Controlling Fluctuations of Diabetes Blood Glucose, Healing and Preventing Nerve Damage
with
Baby's Milk

by
Leonida Lidman

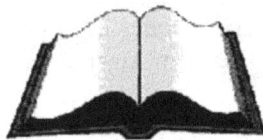

CCB Publishing
British Columbia, Canada

Controlling Fluctuations of Diabetes Blood Glucose, Healing and Preventing Nerve Damage with Baby's Milk

Copyright ©2002, 2004, 2005, 2009 by Leonida Lidman
ISBN-13   978-1-926585-63-5
Second Edition

Library and Archives Canada Cataloguing in Publication

Lidman, Leonida, 1938-
Controlling fluctuations of diabetes blood glucose, healing and preventing nerve damage with baby's milk / written by Leonida Lidman – 2nd ed.
ISBN 978-1-926585-63-5
Also available in electronic format.
1. Diabetes--Diet therapy. 2. Blood sugar. 3. Infant formulas.
4. Lidman, Leonida, 1938- --Health. 5. Diabetics--United
States--Biography. 6. Diabetes--Popular works. I. Title.
RC662.L54 2009   616.4'620654   C2009-907023-5

Publisher: CCB Publishing
             British Columbia, Canada
             www.ccbpublishing.com

DEDICATIONS

SPECIAL THANKS AND APPRECIATION TO:

Professor Jennie C. Brand-Miller, Ph.D

World's Foremost Authority on Glycemic Index Food Values; Founder, Director Nutritional Research Laboratory, University of Sydney, Australia for her most valuable contribution that led to the solution of this author's life-threatening problem of insulin fluctuations.

This work is also lovingly dedicated
to my grandchildren:

Matthew Kennedy, Jr.
and
Aimee Rabino

who inspired me to write my experience with diabetes

and to my husband, Walter J. Lidman
for his emotional and material support
as well as to
all persons afflicted with diabetes

TABLE OF CONTENTS

INTRODUCTION

This book tells graphically the constant pain and life-threatening complications related to Type 2 Diabetes which has afflicted the author for the past 18 years.

Diabetes has no known cure. It is a global scourge that has emerged as the biggest national and worldwide crippler and killer faster than major illnesses such as heart disease and cancer. ("The Stealth Epidemic", The New York Times, January 9, 2006).

The most recent report on diabetes by the U.S. Center for Disease Control in 2000 revealed 21,000,000 Americans with diabetes and predicted that 41,000,000 more will get it. The World Health Organization reported 121,000,000 afflicted and predicted that 266,900,000 more will get it worldwide.

Typically, complications of Type 2 Diabetes set in years before any symptoms appear and before they are diagnosed. (Richard Kahn, Ph.D., Chief Scientific and Medical Officer, American Diabetes Association)

These reports from the U.S. Center for Disease Control and from the American Diabetes Association confirm that medical complications that diabetes sets off attack every major organ, causing severe nerve damage along with painful swelling of fingers, joints and knuckles; muscle aches and pains; painful tingling of the legs and feet; restless legs; wounds that do not heal that lead to amputation; severe imbalance in walking; bladder problems and kidney diseases needing excruciating dialysis.

This book is about controlling Type 2 Diabetes and preventing this crippling nerve damage, preventable pain and destruction of major organs by eating 'healing' or low-glycemic foods; drinking baby's milk formula; regular exercise and taking prescribed medication. All are paramount in the control and prevention of this killer disease.

CHAPTER I

The Urgent Phone Call about My Diabetes and the Medical Treatment that Followed

Prior to being diagnosed as diabetic in 1991, I suffered frequent urination; excessive thirst; blurry vision; fatigue; frequent indigestion; diarrhea; profuse sweating at night even in cold weather; swollen knuckles; pinpricks on my hands, legs and feet which felt like bugs crawling inside my skin. My former family physician, Dr. Antonio Loreno, called this "tingling sensation" and advised rubbing liniments and applying a hot water bag massage on my legs when the liniments didn't work and elevating my legs when asleep. This only worked for a few hours but never completely relieved my discomfort.

For excessive urination and thirst, Dr. Loreno told me to avoid sweets, salty and fatty foods. For extreme fatigue, he prescribed daily over the counter vitamins; a refreshing warm bath before sleeping; avoiding alcohol (which I never drink) and caffeine from coffee which I drink excessively.

He ordered a blood test which showed the onset of diabetes. He referred me to a diabetes specialist, Dr. Muriel Levy-Kern, who classified the blood test result as "diabetes in limbo" since the blood sugar level was not high enough to be classified as diabetes and not low enough to assure that diabetes was not present.

It was very comforting when Dr. Loreno advised that I could avoid diabetes by eating no sweets, no salty or fatty foods and exercise like walking around the block.

In the summer of 1991 an urgent phone call alerted me to a very dangerous medical condition.

Dr. Thomas Klepacki of the Prudential Insurance Company advised me that my husband's life insurance application on my behalf was denied.

Sensing that I was nervous and defensive, he urged me to write his address: Prudential Insurance; Eastern Medical Operation at Fort Washington, PA. 19034 with his phone number 215-754-2401. It was a very unusual call. When he urged me to rush to the emergency room of our local hospital and tell my family physician to call him. I nervously replied, "I am not going to any emergency room and won't call my family physician unless you, Dr. Klepacki, tell me why."

After a few seconds hesitation, Dr. Klepacki said, "I am not allowed to give professional advice even though I am a medical doctor, since my work with Prudential is insurance. Your blood sample taken by the nurse from Prudential showed a dangerously high urine glucose level of 9 mg/dl and blood glucose of 652 mg/dl. I called you because this information alarmed me. I suspect diabetes." He volunteered to wait an hour in his office so as not to miss my physician's call.

What a very kind and caring man!

He continued pleading, "Mrs. Lidman, please go to the hospital. If you are unable to contact your family doctor, the emergency room physician will contact him for you. But please. PLEASE. Go to the hospital. Ask someone to drive you. You could lose consciousness. Your vision could blur."

After I murmured, "Thank you," he wished me well and hung up.

Immediately my husband rushed me to the emergency room of Bayshore Hospital in Holmdel, New Jersey.

The triad nurse recorded the information that Dr. Klepacki advised. Another took my blood sample and told me the results would be available in two hours. She led me to an improvised waiting room and gave me an oxygen tube as I lay in the bed.

I must have slept because when I awoke, the wall clock read 2 A.M.

How??? I got here after 5P.M.

I dimly recognized Dr. Loreno and Dr. Levy-Kern in their white doctor's coats standing at my bedside.

"What time is it?" I asked.

Neither answered.

"Did I pass out?"

Neither answered.

Gently, Dr. Loreno filled me in. He introduced the nursing staff who specialized in diabetic care. "You're on the fourth floor of the diabetic department. Go back to sleep."

Dr. Levy-Kern added, "I'll go home to get some sleep too."

Go back to sleep? How? I was wide awake.

How did I get to the fourth floor?

"Go back to sleep," said the nurse who took my blood.

"Go back to sleep," said another nurse who came for a urine sample.

"Hello, you look better," said yet another nurse who took my blood pressure and pushed a thermometer inside my mouth, saying, "Under your tongue. Under your tongue," looking at her wristwatch to check my pulse. "There. There. Very good. Very good."

These nurses may be good at their jobs but how are patients supposed to go back to sleep when they wake us up as soon as we fall asleep?

They wake you up to take blood samples; they probe you with stethoscopes; they count your pulse; they shove thermometers under your tongue and demand urine specimens.

The worst place to sleep is a hospital.

Since Dr. Klepacki's frightening phone call and my

hospital stay in 1991, my life had not been normal until 2002 when I noticed a big difference in my energy level. This high level of energy continues to this date, 2009, after I made and followed my own diet plan (menu) based on the Glycemic Index Food information in the Glucose Revolution Books, suggested by Dr. Jennie Brand-Miller. I had more pep and a wonderful sense of well-being. My strength increased and I felt energized and ready to do all the endless household chores.

What made this huge difference?

"The food!"*

During my four day hospitalization, Dr. Loreno, Dr. Levy-Kern, a social worker and a dietician, along with the nursing staff kept track of my blood glucose. Too high or too low is dangerous.

To perform blood tests I was taught to prick the tip of my finger with a small lancet which holds a tiny needle; place a drop of blood on a reagent strip and insert it into a small digital machine which reports the glucose level. This taught me to be aware when my blood sugar rose above 160/180 mg/dl. The urine often contained white spots which are dried splashes of glucose-filled urine in the toilet bowl. I looked for this and noted it keenly in my daily logs.

This information helps my physician determine whether

---

* Author's note: "The food" to which the author refers is "healing foods" in the Glycemic Index in Chapter III and "baby's milk" in Chapter V.

my diet went awry; whether there is a need to readjust my oral medication; whether other types of tests are needed; whether I should be tested for albumin.

The social worker concentrated on my mental health – a major diabetic issue involving depression; suppressed anger; personality changes; mood swings; and the impact of all these on me every day.

She added the availability of health professionals, should the need arise.

I felt like a bewildered animal who lost its way. My diabetes felt like a death sentence.

A nurse educator visited me daily and gave me free diabetic testing supplies and equipment. She showed me how to take blood and urine samples and how to record the results in a special self-testing log. My reluctance irritated her since I cannot stand needles pricking me, let alone the sight of blood, especially my own.

According to the nurse diabetic educator, I must be keenly aware of my blood glucose level every day without fail. Here is what I learned.

WHEN BLOOD GLUCOSE (mg/dl) is:	COMMENTS
Below 70 mg/dl	I must follow treatment plan for low blood sugar.

70-120 mg/dl fasting blood glucose	This glucose level is ideal. No cause for alarm.
70-140 mg/dl fasting blood glucose	This glucose level is acceptable.
100-140 mg/dl blood glucose after meals (1 ½ to 2 hours)	This glucose level is ideal.
120-180 mg/dl blood glucose after meals (1 ½ to 2 hours)	This glucose level is acceptable.
Above 200 mg/dl	Glucose level is not acceptable. I must call my physician and report this.
Above 240 mg/dl	I must test for ketones. If ketones are present, or if my blood sugar does not return to normal in 2 days, I must contact my physician.

I learned so much from my hospital stay and from consultation with Dr. Levy-Kern, Dr. Loreno and hospital nurse-educator that I feel compelled to share my experience. The knowledge I gained about Type 2 diabetes from these skilled professionals guided me well. For instance, I was able to accept gradually that diabetes, a lifelong condition that has no known cure, is caused by increased glucose in the blood, by insufficient insulin production or by inability of the insulin to work effectively.

In the beginning, none of this was easy to understand. When I was dangerously ill with this life-threatening condition, all I wanted to know is when I would get well and how soon.

It was mentally challenging to comprehend how food is broken down into glucose, the body's main source of energy; that when insulin is absent, reduced or not effective, glucose cannot be transported to the cells for energy. When this happens, glucose builds up in the blood. This high blood glucose level causes diabetes.

The nurse educator and Dr. Levy-Kern both said that meal planning, physical exercise, medication, stress management and knowledge about diabetes all help blood glucose levels to return to or remain normal.

According to these professionals, diabetes is not contagious. Obesity and heredity precipitate it. Since I am never overweight, obesity did not play a role. The susceptibility to diabetes is passed from generation to generation through the genes but not in any predictable pattern. Dr. Levy-Kern said that heredity played a part in my being diabetic. I was diagnosed with Type 2 (non-insulin dependent diabetes mellitus) due to heredity since my father was diabetic and passed away due to its many complications.

Dr. Levy-Kern emphasized the necessity to watch for high blood sugar (HYPERGLYCEMIA) and low blood sugar (HYPOGLYCEMIC). I was given written information on what to expect and how to detect symptoms. Here's the information:

KNOW THE DIFFERENCE BETWEEN HIGH BLOOD SUGAR AND LOW BLOOD SUGAR

HIGH BLOOD SUGAR: (HYPERGLYCEMIA)

Symptoms noticed within hours to several days:

- increased thirst and frequent urination

- large amounts of blood sugar

- ketones in urine

- weakness, pains in stomach, aching all over

- heavy-labored breathing

- loss of appetite, nausea, vomiting

- fatigue

LOW BLOOD SUGAR (HYPOGLYCEMIA)

Symptoms noticed within minutes to hours:

- cold sweats

- dizziness, headaches

- blurred vision

- inability to awaken

- grouchiness

- personality change

WHAT TO DO:

- call doctor immediately

- take fluids without sugar if able to swallow
- test blood sugar frequently
- test urine for ketones

- call doctor

WHAT TO DO:

- take 2 glucose tablets or food containing sugar (orange juice, regular soda)
- check blood sugar level
- do not give insulin

- do not give anything by mouth if unconscious

CAUSES

- not enough insulin
- too much food
- infection, fever, illness

- emotional stress

CAUSES

- too much insulin
- not enough food
- overly strenuous exercise
- delayed meal

For high blood sugar, Dr. Levy-Kern and Dr. Loreno strongly advised me to monitor the blood sugar and urine ketone levels. Urine testing for ketones can be done at home with test kits from the pharmacy. I prefer to have my ketone tests done in a laboratory to make sure there is no possible kidney problem. It is hard enough to have diabetes, and it is deadly when kidneys are affected.

Long ago my father said, "No one dies from diabetes, but diabetic complications will surely get you." He should know. He died from diabetes complications of the kidneys, circulation problems and high blood pressure.

Prior to being released from the hospital, the nurse educator enrolled me in a month-long diabetes self-management course. Family members were encouraged to attend. The course included:

- general information supported by numerous pamphlets of information from various sources
- blood glucose monitoring
- oral hypoglycemic
- ketone testing
- hygiene, nutrition and meal planning
- stress management
- behavior medication
- group discussion

Meeting with other diabetics and their families helped the diabetic team to assist me to control my blood sugar and to understand personality changes and mood swings that impact my husband and children and inspire them to be more patient and tolerant.

RECOMMENDATIONS FOR KETONE TESTING

Persons with Type 2 Non-Insulin Dependent Diabetes should call their doctor when:

1. blood sugar is greater than 240 mg/dl and ketones are positive in the urine

2. the blood sugar has increased over the past 12 hours and tests show the presence of ketones.

Two kidneys in the back of our spine above the waistline filter blood flow through tiny capillaries. High levels of ketones in urine warn of possible kidney problems. Kidney complications include fatigue, lower back pain and light burning sensation while urinating.

To determine whether my diabetes is affecting my kidneys, my physician recommends microalbumin laboratory tests at least once a year.

When I experience light burning sensations while voiding, I usually drink cranberry cocktail juice for 2-3 days. When the painful sensation does not go away, doctors prescribe antibiotics to treat possible infections in the urinary tract. Cranbury juice is now my regular beverage. I take a half glass at least once daily.

Oral medication was prescribed twice daily which, in

recent years, was reduced to one tablet twice daily. I take my prescription to this day.

In the beginning, I was instructed to monitor my blood sugar every four hours, six times a day. Even at night I had to prick my fingers twice – I had to – even though I had difficulty getting back to sleep.

Pricking my fingers – forefinger; middle finger; ring finger – so many times produced ugly calluses. Sometimes no blood came out, since the skin had hardened. With the needle so small I feared it would break and embed the tip under my skin, so I often had to prick myself twice, sometimes thrice. I abhor pricking myself, even though the needle is small and the pain is bearable. Nonetheless, I cannot stand the sight of blood, especially my own.

Each month Dr. Levy-Kern smiled when she read my logbook showing a much lower blood sugar level than the previous month; or frowned when the glucose level rose.

In addition to daily pricking my fingertips, Dr. Levy-Kern ordered a hospital glycated hemoglobin blood test, or HbAIC, which gave a three to four month average blood sugar reading.

She explained that HbAIC tests measure how much sugar is attached to protein in the red blood cells, which have a life-span of three months – hence the three-month averaging of sugar level in the blood as determined in the laboratory.

I discovered that pricking a few times daily is truly meaningful. In the morning before breakfast my reading is mostly low; after lunch my blood sugar surges higher than expected. Before dinner the sugar level can be normal but after dinner, the glucose also surges within two hours.

In the beginning it annoyed me no end to prick my fingers. I realized, however, doing so made me aware of the fluctuating glucose level which I had to avoid and control to prevent complications that could damage my body organs. The fluctuations of my glucose levels in different hours of the day made me realize that pricking my fingers just once daily was a grave risk. I began to appreciate the value, even though it depressed me immensely.

By this time I had a new family physician, Dr. Thomas Scuderi, who also treats diabetics. I explained my feelings to him. After examining me and reading my logbook which reflected stable glucose levels, he finally reduced the finger-pricking to three times a day; then twice a day. However, even pricking myself once a day became exasperating for me. I simply couldn't do it any more.

He finally agreed for me to prick my fingers three times a week – once every other day – on condition that on those days, my glucose level remain stable and that I strictly observe my Food Exchange Plan. I gratefully agreed.

As ordered, I strictly observed my food intake, dutifully took my prescribed medications and exercised moderately as required.

When I detected low blood sugar (hypoglycemia), I immediately pricked my finger. When the meter showed low blood sugar, confirming my suspicion, I took two glucose tablets which I keep with me everywhere I go during the day and on my side of the bed at night. Their melting in my mouth reduces my weakness and stops my profuse cold sweats and makes me feel warm again. Low glucose (hypoglycemic) makes me hungry and thirsty but the glucose tablets reduce my weakness and recharge my energy. As a result, I could easily go to the kitchen for toast, unsalted crackers and a half glass of orange juice.

During hypoglycemia attacks which happen often in my sleep, I can hardly get out of bed to walk to the kitchen for those unsalted crackers and orange juice.

How do I detect hypoglycemia when I am deeply asleep? Cold perspiration soaks my pajamas and wakes me up.

When I continue feeling cold all over even after taking glucose tablets and wearing extra clothing, I call Dr. Scuderi who usually asks me to report to his clinic for observation.

When I detect high blood glucose (hyperglycemia) by heavy-labored breathing when I am not doing anything; nausea; body aches, I immediately prick my fingertips to see if my blood sugar rose very high. When it does, I immediately take water preferably, followed by a couple of hours of rest and sleep. When I wake up feeling my blood sugar is still high, I prick my fingertips to see how high. I always make a doctor's appointment when the blood sugar remains high. On a few occasions while under observation at Dr. Scuderi's clinic when my blood sugar remains high (over 250 mg/dl), I was given insulin injection which lowered my blood glucose in one to two hours, after which I felt fine again.

Hyperglycemia (high blood sugar) happens over hours and days. It gives you time to observe symptoms and call for help.

Hypoglycemia (low blood sugar) happens fast, leaving minutes to an hour to attend to it. Unattended low blood glucose causes coma or death but it is preventable. Low blood sugar is more dangerous than high blood sugar. The danger of low blood sugar is the main reason I refuse to take the mildest sleeping pills during nights when sleep eludes me. What if my blood sugar went dangerously low? I might not wake up at all.

Hyperglycemia happens over hours and days, giving me 24 hours to observe my symptoms and to call my physician or rush to the emergency room when my blood sugar does not go down to an acceptable level after all the precautions detailed in this book have been observed.

Both high and low blood sugar are dangerous when neglected. My response to both is eternal vigilance. My body warns me. Testing my glucose level confirms those warnings mentioned in this book and I heed them.

During a monthly consultation in the earlier years, my diabetic specialist assumed, correctly, that I had been diabetic before I was medically diagnosed. Therefore, very high blood sugar for years, which led to the phone call from Dr. Klepacki, possibly caused nerve damage or diabetic neuropathies which caused the painful tingling in my hands, legs, thighs and all-over aches and pains.

My family physician and diabetic specialist, in consultation with each other, referred me for a general physical examination, consisting of more X-rays; magnetic resonance imaging (MRI); ultrasound of my arms, shoulders, legs, eyes, ears, nose, throat and thyroid glands; urinalysis and cholesterol to discover the causes of my aches and pains and possible undiagnosed illnesses.

Those exams revealed no organ damage. However, my diabetic specialist concluded that my aches and pains were due to nerve damage in the periphery of my legs, brought on by my diabetes. Neuropathies are difficult to treat, much less prevent when patients don't fully cooperate. "There she goes again," I thought ruefully, biting my lips to prevent myself from arguing.

I knew what she meant. She meant that my aches and pains or nerve damage were because I stopped pricking my fingertips 4 to 6 times daily. She argued against reducing those prickings as allowed by Dr. Scuderi to once a day even when my logbook consistently showed a stable glucose.

I believe that these aches and pains had been with me for a long time before I was diagnosed as diabetic.

How can these neuropathies be prevented now by pricking my fingertips?

Why won't she just remedy my problems?

I just suffered in silence morosely.

CHAPTER II

Exercise

My family physician and diabetic specialist could not overemphasize the importance of regular exercise, light or moderate, and especially walking even only 20 minutes around the block to prevent leg muscles from stiffening and to avert nerve damage to the periphery of the legs.

How did nerve damage affect my legs before I was diagnosed with diabetes if exercise would avert it? I did a lot of walking from the house to the bus stop and back home three blocks away while commuting to work. There was no public transportation near Hazlet, where I live. People in neighboring areas catch the New Jersey Transit train in the next town. Trains that stop at the Hazlet station pick up passengers from every little station. One cannot ride these trains and arrive on time for work. There were buses that went mostly to New York City, but they pass the highway one mile away. I used to work in Newark, New Jersey. Going there by bus was very cumbersome. From New York I had to take a bus to Jersey City which came every half hour, then wait twenty minutes in Journal Square for the bus to Newark.

To avoid this hassle, we commuters from Hazlet petitioned the Academy Bus Company to provide service to Newark. A single bus was provided from Hazlet at 6:15

A.M. and from Newark at 5:45 P.M.

In Newark, the bus dropped us near the Public Service Electric and Gas Co. From there I walked four blocks, taking the shortcut through Military Park to my office. To me, this was a lot of walking, especially during winter and bad weather. Inside, I negotiated three flights of stairs instead of riding the ancient, creaking elevator which made me fear for my safety. If walking 20 minutes daily would prevent my leg muscles from stiffening, yes, I would do it. It should be easy. But was it?

Since I was prematurely retired from employment when I was diagnosed with uncontrolled diabetes, and suffering severe aches and pains, I hardly had to walk any more. I rode everywhere with my husband to go food shopping, to run errands, to shop at malls, and everywhere. To my surprise, the recommended 20 minute walk was a struggle. It was shocking to find that my feet wouldn't carry me. My legs were stiff as a walking cane that wouldn't bend. My feet hurt inside the softest walking shoes while attempting to negotiate the paved surface of the sidewalk.

It pricked my pride to realize that I couldn't walk straight any more. In my younger days, I walked an imaginary straight line that gave bounce to my gait. Now, every step seemed to throw my legs off balance. It was ridiculous just trying to do what was natural and inborn. I had to stop and rest every few minutes and pant for breath. What was so natural since birth, like breathing and walking, was now frustrating. I could hardly negotiate, let alone walk, on uncarpeted surfaces.

When did this start? I had very few problems walking around the house, but I had trouble climbing the stairs. My doctor said that walking on carpeted floors cushioned my feet and legs. But sidewalks, no matter how level they appear, have uneven bumps which we hardly detect, and which my legs can no longer handle. It became more and more apparent that my physical functions were rapidly deteriorating. This was not easy to admit and accept. I made excuses not to walk around the block.

My granddaughter, Aimee, five years old at the time, noticed. One summer she suggested some gardening like we used to do, pulling weeds from around my flowering plants, planting tomatoes, beans and corn in the backyard. I replied that it was a waste of time, since rabbits ate all our vegetables the past summer, and watering the grass and garden was a waste of water. "But Grandma," Aimee pleaded, "didn't we plant those vegetables to feed the rabbits and squirrels and birds?"

I ran out of excuses. Someone in the family must have told Aimee. That summer, Aimee begged me to get out of the house, walk around the block, or simply visit the neighbor's dog, with which she became friendly. When she noticed that my legs were unsteady and needed rest, she would pull me slowly under the shade of trees. As the slow walk around the block became routine, Aimee's sharp instinct determined when I had to rest and when it was Okay to resume our walk. As we continued walking, she held my hand

20

soothingly, whispering, "Come, Grandma, don't be afraid. I won't let you fall."

Oh! How astutely she sensed my unexpressed fear.

Listening to her made me smile as I remembered when she was just learning to walk, and I had coaxed her to walk to me, one step at a time, "Come, Aimee, don't be afraid. I won't let you fall."

There were so many of those bright, joyful moments with sweet little Aimee, who is not so 'little' at this writing. In substance, Aimee taught me, without knowing, not to shrink from what I must face, even pain.

No matter the never ending aches and pains in my feet and leg muscles; no matter how humiliating it was being seen walking around the block unsteadily, supported by a little girl holding my hand with her tiny hand; no matter how hard to accept that old age and ill health had crept up on me too soon; my legs responded to Aimee's constant encouragement. "Walk, Grandma. Walk. When I go to kindergarten, I hope you walk me there." The Hazlet Pre-School, kindergarten and elementary school is three minutes from our house. It took me seventeen minutes one way. But I did walk Aimee to school a few times. I could not disappoint her.

On other occasions, when my husband came home early from his school 37 miles away, he joined Aimee and me to walk in the early evenings. I have been walking around the block, wincing and gritting my teeth. During winter the cold exacerbates the pain, so I merely walk around the house for my exercise.

Spring, Summer and Fall I walked in parking lots of the nearby school, the library and inside the malls where my husband drove me for my needed exercise.

Yet, despite the many years of walking and exercising as the doctor advised, my legs remain weak, wobbly and in pain. I can only wear the softest flat shoes, purchased from catalogs which specialize in shoes and slippers for people with special needs. I continued walking so very slowly and carefully to avoid stepping on uneven surfaces or to prevent my feet from touching objects on the sidewalk.

In 2003, after about six months of taking "the food", the subject of this little book, I began to feel gradual improvement in my legs and steps. Slowly my walk became steady and the pain less and less. At present I can walk more steadily and normally than I've been able in many years.

The following pages are pointers about EXERCISE from a manual from Bayshore Community Hospital of Holmdel, New Jersey, which I copied verbatim, and which I hope will prove useful to others who experience similar problems to mine. However, the only exercise I was able to do from this list is walking, slowly at first, as described here.

DIABETES CONTROL AND EXERCISE

How effective exercise is to the metabolism of a person with diabetes is determined by the amount of insulin available, the degree of diabetes control and the hydration. Theoretically, a person with well-controlled diabetes, whose insulin and food are in proper balance, can handle exercise as well as someone without diabetes. If control is poor, there are significant differences in metabolism.

When diabetes is only under fair control, rather than good control, the body will run out of glucose fuels. It will start to burn free fatty acids, which produce ketones. This is one reason why you never exercise if your blood sugar is over 240 mg/dl unless approved by your physician.

With very poor control, the problem described above is even worse. Blood glucose levels are high, but the lack of insulin prevents the glucose from getting into the cells where it can be metabolized for energy. The liver thinks the body needs more glucose, so it starts pouring more glucose into the blood, causing the blood sugar to go higher. The body keeps using free fatty acids for fuel which produce ketones. The end result is high blood sugar and high ketone levels.

SELF BLOOD GLUCOSE
MONITORING AND EXERCISE

To find out how exercise affects you, test blood sugar before and after exercising. Testing helps you know if you should change your meal plan or medication. Exercise can affect blood sugar for up to 24 hours or more after an activity.

TEST YOUR BLOOD SUGAR:

- when exercising longer than usual and you do not feel well. Stop and rest.
- when beginning a new exercise program or changing to a new one.
- after completing exercise and one hour later. If your blood glucose is dropping, eat a snack and check it later to make sure it is still not dropping.
- when exercising in the evening. Check before bedtime. Always be cautious. Blood sugar may drop too low during sleep.

DO NOT EXERCISE IF:

- blood sugar is above 240 mg/dl unless your doctor has given the approval

- blood sugar is below 100 mg/dl. Delay exercise and eat a snack. Follow the suggestions listed.

THREE STAGES OF EXERCISE

There are three stages of exercise. Each stage is important each time you exercise.

WARMUP: Gets your muscles ready for exercise. Warmup should consist of 5 to 10 minutes of stretching, flexing and rotation exercises such as walking slowly, etc.

This period gets your heart and muscles ready for harder work. Warmups slowly increase your heart rate and loosen muscles and ligaments to prevent soreness or injury.

AEROBIC STAGE: Actual exercise time. Eventually you should work up to 20 to 45 minutes. To achieve maximum benefits, this phase should be at least 20 minutes.

There are three components of the aerobic stage:

1. INTENSITY: effort or how hard you exercise.

2. DURATION: how long you exercise at one session.

3. FREQUENCY: how often you exercise

COOLDOWN STAGE: slowing down the activity and gradually bringing your heart rate back to normal. Slow down your activity before stopping completely. This period should be 5 to 10 minutes long.

DO NOT STOP EXERCISE ABRUPTLY!

Cooldown can be continuous slow walking or stretching, flexing and rotation.

Exercising for long periods of time can also change light exercise into moderate exercise, which is aerobic.

ACTIVITIES

LIGHT	MODERATE	INTENSE
Walking	Brisk walking	Running
Golf	Slow jogging	Cross-Country
Slow skating	Swimming	Skiing
Housework	Aerobic Class	Fast biking
Leisure	Tennis	Football
Canoeing	Water skiing	Hockey
Badminton		Intense Aerobic Class

FOR MAXIMUM AEROBIC BENEFIT:

- Increase to moderate or intense exercise
- Continuously rhythmic in nature

Start slowly as you begin your exercise program over days, weeks or months. Gradually increase the pace.

Whatever exercise you choose, try to exercise your whole body. For example, if you are walking, swing your arms. Keep your back straight, head up and breathe deeply.

If your doctor approves, gradually increase to an aerobic activity. A moderate pace benefits even more. However, an intense pace if for those who are fit and who have the approval of their physician.

- Increase the heart rate to 70-85% maximum
- 20 minutes at maximum heart rate
- 3 to 5 times per week

Here is a simple formula to figure your heart rate:

220 – your age = Maximum heart rate

Maximum heart rate x 60% - 80% target heart rate

Example: John is 50 years old

220 – 50 = 170 maximum heart rate

170 x .60 = minimum heart rate

170 x .80 – 136 maximum heart rate

Ask your doctor what your heart rate should be during the peak of your exercise.

You should learn to take your pulse rate. Your doctor or diabetes educator can help you.

EXERCISE TIMES

- Exercise the same time each day if possible. This allows you to balance your exercise with meals and medication.

- Exercise one to two hours after a meal. This is generally when blood sugar is highest and risk of low blood sugar is reduced.

- Exercise should be done when insulin or diabetes pills are not "peaking" (working their best).

- If you exercise in the evening, you may have to add fruit or milk to your bedtime snack.

- Be aware of the potential for low blood sugar during sleep if you exercise in the evening.

- If you are changing the times of your exercise, check with your physician so that changes in medication or meal plans can be made.

DURATION

When you begin your exercise program, do not tire yourself. You may only be able to exercise 5 minutes with a 1 to 2 minute warmup and cooldown.

As you become more fit, you can gradually work longer periods. To achieve a moderate rate, exercise for 20 minutes at 70% to 85% of your maximum heart rate. The warm-ups and cooldown will be 5 to 10 minutes.

To lose weight, you should exercise longer rather than harder.

If you are fit and your blood sugars are under good control, you do not need to limit your exercise sessions.

Remember to eat extra snacks as needed during activity to balance long periods of exercise.

FREQUENCY

To reap the maximum benefits of exercising, be consistent. Exercise 3 to 5 times each week if possible. This also allows the body to rest between sessions.

Do not give up if you miss a week or two. Just begin

your routine from the start, not from where you left off.

If you need to lose weight, you should exercise about 5 times a week and follow a weight loss meal plan.

Plan other activities for bad weather especially during winter months such as mall walking, indoor swimming or calisthenics.

In 2007 while watching a Home Shopping TV Network, an advertisement appeared about a portable foot exerciser. I ordered one immediately.

This portable exerciser is lightweight with its own storage bag which can be taken anywhere. It can be pedaled while sitting, drinking coffee, watching TV or reading the newspapers or, in my case, watching cars driving by or bird-watching while sitting on my porch. This is why this exerciser is called "walking while you sit". It was I who added this portable foot exerciser to the recommended walking around the block and calisthenics.

CHAPTER III

Controlling Fluctuations of Blood Glucose from Sudden Sugar High to Sugar Low

While walking to exercise my legs in the corridors of the diabetic section of the hospital, I observed other patients on wheelchairs with amputated legs in bandages and others in walkers, hardly able to ambulate. Looking pained, one gestured, pointing to his backside and said, "Kidney surgery."

"My Lord," I prayed, "please don't let me die with painful organ damage. Please allow me to live a fruitful life and die peacefully in my sleep."

It was a shock to see so many people sick like me in the same corridor, adding to the turmoil going through me when the doctors said I have diabetes far enough to need medication. It won't go away by mere diet and exercise.

In 1992, in addition to prescribed medication, a dietician developed for me an 1800 calorie meal food exchange plan.

This plan guided me daily on what to eat, when to eat, and what amount to eat. If I ate too much at one meal or ate meals too close together, my blood sugar might get too high. If I ate too little or skipped a meal, my blood sugar might become dangerously low.

The meal plan included three meals a day: snacks of unsalted crackers and a cup of nonfat milk with no sugar or with Sweet-and-Low at 10:30 A.M. The plan recommended another snack at 3:00 P.M. with a nighttime snack again of unsalted crackers and milk and jell-o. The two snacks during the day and the other one before bedtime were necessary because I was employed while my diabetes was uncontrolled and I had to maintain my energy level to do my job.

The individualized meal plan provided a nutritionally balanced diet through six basic food groups:

> starches/bread
>
> vegetables
>
> milk
>
> meat and poultry
>
> fat
>
> fruits

Each food group, I was told, contains the same nutritional value of calories in the portion size listed. For example, one slice of bread = 1/2 cup of pasta = 1/3 cup of rice.

Within each group I could substitute food items within the groups as long as I adhered to the proper portion size. I could not exchange food items between groups. For example, I could not substitute a bread item for a fruit item. This very strictly-controlled diet takes a lot of discipline. Often I resented it. Sometimes I broke the rules. The muscle aches and pains that followed warned me severely to discipline myself.

To prevent heart disease I had to strictly limit the amount and types of fat in my diet. Saturated fat or fats from animal sources increased bad cholesterol which can cause heart disease. This restriction is challenging because I love fried pork; pork adobo cooked in soy sauce, onions, vinegar; chicken and shrimp cooked in coconut milk which is highly saturated with fats.

However, a recent study in *Health and Healing Newsletter* indicated that the saturated fat in coconut milk contains good cholesterol. This becomes bad only when it is denatured through heat and chemicals. This good news enabled me to cook chicken, shrimp and vegetables in coconut milk as Asians do.

The dietician recommended lean meat like skinless chicken; turkey; fish; beef in small portions, as well as skim milk and skim milk products and light salad dressing. Food should be baked, roasted, broiled or grilled rather than fried. Fortunately, I am here in the United States where food choices are extremely plentiful. All I needed was self-control with my diet. I was strictly cautioned not to overeat. But it was not easy.

Meticulously following the Food Exchange Plan day after day for years was a constant struggle. Consistently measuring cup after measuring cup of this and that food; determining 1 oz., 3 oz., 4 oz. of carbohydrates and protein portions; 1/2 tsp. by gram of fat depressed me, making me feel like a slave to a diet plan. For many years I was unable to think about anything but my food intake.

When I complained, my doctor admonished: "Unrestricted amounts, especially of sweet, salty and fatty foods cause complications that could kill you. So grit your teeth and follow your diet. It's for your own good."

Although I learned to accept the benefits of the Food Exchange Plan and the danger of not following it, I cheated on a few occasions. At Filipino parties, it was extremely hard to resist Philippine foods I knew since childhood, cooked in heavy coconut syrup, syrup from sugar cane such as rice cakes; coconut gel; coconut meat from mutant coconut; palm fruits and other sweet flans. Equally tempting are Philippine cakes with desiccated coconut and bread from arrowroot (a kind of tuber that grows underground like carrots). There are also pastries and Danish and cakes in the pastry and frozen food section of U.S supermarkets. All are mouth-watering and tempting.

Each time I sampled these foods, especially when I went for second helpings, I felt my face and lips swell as if injected with novocaine. Why? I merely sampled them.

"But you sampled a few and they add up," my husband said.

Those swellings, accompanied by muscle aches and pains, were grave warnings not to ignore doctor's advice and to stick to the portion sizes in my daily menu, no matter how tempted I was.

Yet, even when I adhered to the strict daily diet in the menu plan, my blood sugar fluctuated often, most times with very high readings in my glucose meter monitor, followed by very low readings which gave me chills all over with little warning during the day and at night.

The rollercoaster fluctuation of my blood sugar (glucose) has been a problem I dread constantly. What am I to do?

The doctor's advice has been the same: eat only in moderation. "I bet you are overeating. Don't eat the wrong foods. Dissolve one or two glucose tablets in the mouth when your sugar is very low or drink a small glass of orange juice. Call my office or go to the emergency room. The hospital resident doctor will call me."

I kept running to my doctor's office with almost the same complaint. He recommended me again to a diabetic specialist who pricked my fingertips each visit, read the blood sugar count in the monitor and compared the reading from the logbook of daily readings each day of the month.

The specialist told me to keep a journal of the food I ate each day; when the blood glucose went up or down; what I did during the day; whether I was stressed; my daily activities to the minutest detail, in addition to maintaining the logbook of glucose readings.

"Stress also affects blood fluctuations, you know," advising me to take a short nap during the day, to listen to relaxing music to calm me when feeling stressed out and to take warm baths.

To not be tempted to eat more than recommended in my meal plan and to avoid delicacies, especially sweets that are everywhere in our refrigerator and in the glass cabinet which members of my family bring home for their consumption – is very, very frustrating. Just looking at or seeing those foods made me hungry all the time. I wanted to devour them.

Thus, I drank coffee to assuage my hunger before meals; after each meal and during snacks, adding crackers with more at home and in the office. Thus, I consumed about five to six large cups a day which, I thought, gave me energy to function on the job. But when my physician and diabetic specialist heard this, I thought both would have a stroke.

They ordered me in no uncertain terms to gradually reduce my coffee intake to two medium cups a day or face possible ministroke or even paralysis by overloading my heart with caffeine.

Scared out of my wits (who wants to be paralyzed by a stroke?) I drastically reduced my coffee-drinking in two weeks! Since this was too sudden, I became sluggish, grouchy and nervous. I developed blinding headaches. My doctor recommended over-the-counter medicine.

I remained so drowsy and sluggish at work that I had to skip lunch to get an hour's sleep in the back room of my office. Skipping lunch and/or not eating lunch on time could lead to hypoglycemia (low blood sugar) which is also very dangerous for diabetics.

As a result of my sudden break from coffee, my hands

developed tremors. I could not hold a pen. I could not write reports or type, since my fingers kept sliding from the typewriter. Coupled with blinding headaches, drowsiness and feeling lousy on the job, I felt terrible at not being able to function as well as before. I developed job stress as a result.

At nighttime I had interchanging cold and hot flashes, though my menopause was long past. No amount of thick blankets, nor running hot water bottles all over me could stop the trembling. My doctor called this violent episode "withdrawal from caffeine".

This painful withdrawal from caffeine lasted about two months. Since then, I only have a cup of coffee with plenty of lowfat milk at breakfast. I substitute hot tea (green tea) with lemon for snacks and after supper, which became a ritual after-dinner drink with my husband.

I lost plenty of weight. I looked gaunt and became very thin while my skin wrinkled horribly, especially on my face. I looked very old.

I complained to my doctor constantly about fluctuations of my blood sugar and of feeling hunger all the time, while I demanded a new meal plan with more food in the menu.

"Every patient of mine who is diabetic has problems with blood glucose fluctuations. You are not alone. What I suspect is that you are either overeating or eating foods you are not supposed to eat. Tell me, what have you been doing?" my doctor asked. "Don't talk to me about wrinkles.

We all develop them as we age."

"I already told you about my coffee drinking and I had stopped as you advised. I am following the meal plan you approved. However, I doubled the serving of my vegetables. Those are cooked in plain water with shrimps, drops of lemon juice or tamarind powder. My chicken is skinless, cooked on the grill or baked with drops of lemon to marinate, sprinkled with Ms. Dash to taste and lemon, pepper or when boiled, cooked with lots and lots of green, leafy vegetables, potatoes and ginger or coconut oil. What's wrong with those foods?" He had no answer but promised to call the hospital dietician for information.

On my next visit, my doctor claimed that there was a new hospital dietician who could not make a new meal plan unless he confined me in a hospital and prescribed new blood or other tests which are all out of the question, since my situation could not be classified as emergency and my health insurance will not pay.

When my diabetes specialist read again the new entry in my journal, she immediately dialed my doctor and spoke, upset, to him about her findings, namely:

- there's more potatoes, fried or boiled garnished with other vegetables like yams (sweet potatoes), cheeses and sauces in my menu

- there's corn (white corn, sweet corn, Mexican corn) boiled, fresh or in the can consistently added to the daily diet
- rice of different varieties either boiled or steamed and fried mixed with fried pork, and other vegetables served almost three times a day (even in small portions only)
- plantain and potatoes, either fried or cooked in syrup or rice cakes with shredded coconut or desiccated coconut at snack time

Very upset, the diabetic specialist questioned who advised me to eat those foods in the manner described in my journal.

"I did, but what's wrong with those foods, eaten in very small quantities to solve my constant feeling of hunger?"

"It's those foods eaten and/or included in your diet plan almost daily. Those are not substitutes for items in your menu, but an addition to it that is making you hungry and sicker."

Instead of sitting to explain what problems she found in the foods that I added to the menu that she claimed made me sicker, my diabetes specialist said, "Stop what you are doing immediately. Stick to your old meal plan before it's too late for us to help you," she demanded with frustration in her voice and in her face.

"Set an immediate appointment with your doctor who will explain everything you want to know. I will discuss lengthily with him the reasons you are having so many problems. You may request a detailed written explanation from him."

My self-control and discipline were tested again. It was extremely difficult to return to the 1992 Meal Plan which measured food into 2 tbsps. of this; 1/3 cup of that and 3 ounces of another, especially where the menu did not have rice or potatoes in it.

I was from an agricultural country of rice, potato and root crops-eating people who eat these foods three times a day. Try telling people like me to partake of these food items only once a week in very small portions or to stop eating them altogether – they'll act in disbelief as I did.

I tried with great difficulty to go back to the almost 20-year-old diet plan while I also read newsletters and magazines and subscribed to books about diabetes, diabetic problems and menu plans most of which have high calorie content. Most menus are not for diabetics.

In those readings I came across a term called "glycemic index" and "glycemic load" in foods, which I, a lay person, interpreted to mean eating nutrient-filled foods in small portions only similar to my 1992 Meal Plan, measuring calories tablespoon by tablespoon like the menus of appetizing-looking foods in those magazines and TV advertisements, teaching people to lose weight. I already lost weight and had nothing more to lose and have followed once again my old menu plan in portion sizes with the exception of rice and potatoes in small portions only in my daily food intake. I just will not and can not give them up any more.

The <u>Merriam-Webster Collegiate Dictionary</u>, eleventh edition, defines glycemic index as "a measure of the rate at which ingested food causes the level of glucose in the blood to rise".

What, exactly, does this mean? The sudden rise of my blood sugar has been my problem. Which food causes the sudden rise of blood glucose? All food? The amount of food? I couldn't find the answer in any of those magazines and books, so I kept reading.

The Free Data Information in the Internet cited many studies about glycemic index, but those sources cannot be downloaded and copied because no print of them is available in the Internet since they are copyrighted and permission has to be secured from those sources which I tried, to no avail. I also have to request information from the Copyright Office in Washington, D.C. which cannot grant permission without authorization from authors. Our small local library has no copy of any of these research.

Determined to find which food causes levels of glucose in the blood to rise suddenly so I could help myself and so I could include this information in my manuscript for the book I am planning to publish, my husband and I once more sat at the computer, hoping to find something we could be missing. We could not just give up –– now that I have found a term that sounded very interesting for my own health issues.

When fluctuations in blood sugar suddenly happen – it is truly scary. I could be feeling normal and well ready to do the obligations of the day – when suddenly and unexpectedly I feel ill and in discomfort, accompanied by difficult breathing and sudden weakness. The day's schedule is disrupted. Everything planned for the day stops.

It is especially frightening in the evening while at rest or in my sleep. I wake up chilled and sweating profusely. Rushing to prick my fingertip to find the measure of blood glucose in the digital meter machine either very low or very high is alarming, since early in the day and in the evening blood tests, the results were normal or acceptable.

So, searching the Internet again for sources of missing information, we found a name.

It turned out she is not just a name. Her name is Professor Jennette C. Brand-Miller, Ph.D., the world's foremost authority on Glycemic Index; author of several books on Glucose Revolution. How could we have missed her? Perhaps we gave up too easily. We are accustomed to finding literature/written articles on any information and when we don't find such written literature, we think we will never find it.

"Professor Brand-Miller is BIG, very BIG in her field and very busy as a professor of nutrition in Sydney, Australia, and a founder and director of a Modern Nutritional Research Laboratory; a world lecturer. Would she even read, much less reply to my inquiry?" I murmured softly as my heart sank hopelessly.

"Let's e-mail her," my husband said.

"E-mail! Why not a formal letter of request?"

"We'll e-mail first, then, on Monday we will airmail a letter of request," my husband replied as he proceeded to type an e-mail Saturday, August 29, 2009, 8:34 A.M., U.S. time.

Lo! And behold! I was awe-struck.

Professor Brand-Miller e-mailed back – five hours later, August 29, 1:33 P.M.

"That was fast! Look at the date and time! Unbelievable!" I exclaimed.

"Haven't you heard of the International Time Zone?" my husband replied, happy at my good fortune.

The information sent by Professor Brand-Miller included recommendation to read a glucose revolution book and two volumes of International Tables of Glycemic Index and Glycemic Load which are:

1. Table A-1, Glycemic Index (GI) and Glycemic Load (GL) values determined in subjects with normal glucose: 2008

2. Table A-2, Glycemic Index (GI) and Glycemic Load values determined in subjects with impaired glucose tolerance (diabetes) with small subject numbers in values showing wide variability: 2008

Only Professor Brand-Miller and her associates can fully

explain their research methodology conducted in her laboratory in Sydney. The results of those laboratory tests on the effect of carbohydrates on people with immune deficiencies and others are in the tables A-1 and A-2 and explained in American English in her series of books about New Glucose Revolution such as the three books I read with great interest, namely The New Glucose Revolution Low GI Vegetarian Cookbook; Shopper's Guide to GI Values: 2009 and a book about cooking for those trying to lose weight.

Here is the valuable information I found that pertains to my question about causes of sudden fluctuations in blood glucose level:

1. Glycemic Index (GI) only applies to carbohydrate-rich food. It measures how quickly our body digests carbohydrates; that there are foods rich with high volumes of carbohydrates and foods with low volumes of carbohydrates.

   My misconception before I learned this definition of glycemic index and how carbohydrate food relates to the fluctuation of blood glucose include:

   carbohydrate foods such as bread, rice and other starchy foods have the same or similar value; hence, I did not discriminate, which one negatively affects me as a diabetic. I choose them like I were normal and have no constraint in my food intake. I ate them all in small portions according to my menu plan. But I was doing it the wrong way. I mixed three food exchanges in one or two meals daily.

I was not aware until I read the New Glucose Revolution books that even though I could eat these carbohydrate foods I must choose which rice is the better rice due to low GI content; which bread is a better bread. I must not eat high GI rice with loads of potatoes or vegetable-rich meals, which I did.

When I advised my doctor about the changes I made in my diet, I told him about having double servings of vegetables. He did not object. Now, in the New Glucose Revolution book, I learned that vegetables are classified as carbohydrate-filled food too because they are plant foods which leaves someone like me to again make a choice. Though I know potatoes are carbohydrate food, I treated them as vegetables and mixed them with other vegetables such as green, leafy and orange-colored like squash and sweet potato (yam), all are high-volume GI food. Thus, a double-whammy of carbohydrate food items that does not easily metabolize in the body. Thus, bringing the sudden spike of high blood glucose that made me feel ill.

Another mistake I made for years was serving these high volume carbohydrate foods twice daily at lunch and dinner. I thought all vegetables are healthy and good which it is for normal people with no immune problem in their system. But my readings in the series of New Glucose Revolution books changes all those misconceptions.

Glycemic Index (GI) ranked carbohydrates on the scale of 0 to 100 according to the extent carbohydrate raised blood glucose levels after eating. The American Journal of Clinical

Nutrition Vol. 76. No. 1 (2002) S. 56 and The Shopper's Guide to GI Values: 2009. The American Diabetes Association in 2006 indicated foods with high GI are those which are rapidly digested and absorbed and result in marked fluctuations in blood sugar levels. Low GI foods by virtue of their slow digestion and absorption produce gradual rises in blood sugar and insulin levels.

These explanations did not say which foods have high GI value and which have low GI value.

Dr. Brand-Miller's book, Shopper's Guide to GI Values made a distinction on which foods out of 1250 plus contain low, medium and high carbohydrate values – extremely useful for diabetics like me who has been living with problems of sudden fluctuations of blood glucose.

My 1992 Meal Plan did not have a breakdown of the nutrients of each menu, i.e. Calories per serving; calories from fat; saturated fat; cholesterol; dietary fiber; vitamins; calcium, etc. etc. There is no information about exchanges i.e. percent of starches; percent of carbohydrate; lean meat.

The distinction of which food item to choose among the food items such as which type of white rice is a better choice, whether long jasmine white rice or Uncle Ben's converted white rice? Which type of brown rice is a better choice, Thai brown rice or Uncle Ben's brown rice – information readily available in the illustrations outlined specifically for each food group in the New Glucose Revolution Shopper's Guide to GI Values of about 1250-plus food items.

The information in the Shopper's Guide is very recent with publication date of 2009. Perhaps dieticians of over 20 years ago had scant knowledge of the Glycemic Index of foods.

My 1992 Menu Plan worked for me for almost 18 years but I made my own changes out of a need to address my constant feeling of hunger even though I realize now that the change I made was incorrect, and therefore, exposed me to great risk. Now that this goldmine of Glycemic Low Glucose food comes available to me, it will be my food bible that will never part from me.

Glycemic Load (GL) is a term that measures the amount of ingested carbohydrates per serving.

As explained in the Shopper's Guide of GI Values, page 50, Glycemic Load (GL) is calculated by multiplying the GI value of food by the amount of carbohydrates per serving divided by 100.

Glycemic Load = (GI X Carbohydrate per serving) divided by 100

For example, if you wanted to have an apple for a snack, an apple has a GI of 38 (see table in Shopper's Guide) and one medium apple contains 15 grams of carbohydrate, the glycemic load of the apple snack is (38 X 15) divided by 100 = 6.

If you eat two apples, these two apples would have 30 grams of carbohydrates and the GL of the snack is 12. The

GI doesn't change but the amount of carbohydrate increases because two apples are eaten. Page 50, <u>Shopper's Guide to GI Values</u>: 2009.

Other very valuable information in the New Glucose Revolution is A MUST READ FOR EVERYONE. I only noted and explain here information that pertains to the causes of the sudden fluctuations of my blood glucose and insulin levels.

Other information noted is about:

- Table sugar or sucrose which causes blood glucose level to rise only moderately (less than white bread).

- Consumption of white bread (NOT SUGAR) is most strongly related to the incidence of diabetes.

This above information is contrary to what I heard and practice and told by medical professionals. My father who died of diabetes complications did not touch table sugar to the day he passed away. I was advised not to ingest food cooked with table sugar, even fruits that are sweet.

- Sugar substitute with Saccharine is hundreds of times sweeter than sugar; has no effect on blood glucose level and is not metabolized in the body. The GI of Saccharin is 0 (zero) and calories per gram is 0 (zero).

This is very welcome news to me since my sugar substitute for coffee and tea has been a sweetener with Saccharin.

I would love to present in large print the categories and

rank of each of those food items in The Shoppers' Guide to GI Values, since those tables are in very small print, which is difficult reading for elderly diabetics and those with visual problems. The information in the Shopper's Guide is copyrighted and the copyright law prohibits reproduction. I e-mailed a request to Dr. Brand-Miller to copy in large print the Shopper's Guide so I can incorporate with this book. Dr. Brand-Miller suggested to me to request her publisher. Hence this constraint.

Did I find the answer to the fluctuations of my blood glucose? Yes, indeed. Definitely. The definitive answer is on page 29 of the New Glucose Revolution Vegetarian Diet and I quote:

"Low GI food trickles glucose into the bloodstream, slowly; helping to avoid the roller-coaster ride in blood glucose levels to cycle of "sugar high" followed by "sugar low"

"Elevations in blood glucose after eating high GI food are followed by fluctuations of insulin level. The cells that usually respond to insulin become resistant to signal. This means that glucose hangs around in the bloodstream at higher than normal concentrations where it can damage the cells."

Ever since I created and followed a new menu with low GI food items of carbohydrates, other nutrients and fibers found in the New Glucose Revolution books, I only experience three episodes of fluctuations of blood glucose which is very minimal, since in the past 18 or 20 years,

severe fluctuations to high and low levels of glucose has
been my constant companion which I dreaded. This is a new
experience which is truly life-changing.

It is my hope that in the very near future these
fluctuations in blood sugar can be avoided altogether.

I believe this hope is not far-fetched.

My doctor said, "Diabetes has no cure." Maybe. Yet do
we have to live in constant pain and fear? Can't we aspire to
live long and fruitful lives free of radical changes in the
quality of our lives? I believe I found the answer in the New
Glucose Revolution books which advised that choosing low
GI carbohydrates produces smaller fluctuations in blood
glucose which is one of the secrets to long term health of
both diabetics and pre-diabetics.

I wrote these experiences with my diabetes and share
these with others in the hope that they too may find solutions
to problems of complications this dreaded disease brings.

CHAPTER IV

Long-Term Diabetic Complications

According to the following medical guides: *The Bayshore Hospital Educational Manual, The Merck Medical Guide* and *The Medical Guide of The Reader's Digest,* the major organs which diabetes affects are kidneys, eyes and peripheral nerves. Diabetes can affect them to a very different extent. At times, disease in one tissue may be very advanced while another is spared altogether.

Some terms to help the reader understand this chapter:

- nephropathy: diabetic renal (kidney) disease

- retinopathy: diabetic eye disease

- neuropathy: diabetic nerve damage

Thickening of the membranes of blood vessel tissues is the telltale sign of long-standing diabetes. It is seen in the tissues of the retina, kidneys and nerves. It is also seen in skin, muscle and fat tissues.

DIABETIC RENAL (KIDNEY) DISEASE (NEPHROPATHY)

The relevant information that follows is from a booklet about kidney problems caused by high blood sugar, as released by the National Institute of Diabetes and Digestive and Kidney Disease, Information Clearinghouse, Bethesda, MD. 20591 which recommends that said information be disseminated as widely as possible to the general public. Here is the information.

What do kidneys do?

The kidneys act as filters to clean the blood. They get rid of waste and extra fluid. The tiny filters throughout the kidneys are called *glomeruli* (gloh-MEHR-yoo-lie).

When kidneys are healthy, the *artery* (AR-ter-ee) brings blood and waste from the bloodstream into the kidney. The glomeruli clean the blood. Then waste and extra fluid go out into the urine through the ureter. Clean blood goes out of the kidney and back into the bloodstream through the vein.

HOW TO PREVENT DIABETES
KIDNEY PROBLEMS

- Keep your blood glucose as close to normal as you can.

- Keep your blood pressure below 130/30 to help prevent kidney damage. Blood pressure is written with two numbers separated by a slash. For example: 120/70.

- Ask your doctor what numbers are best for you. If you take blood pressure pills, take them as your doctor tells you. Keeping your blood pressure under control will also slow damage to your eyes, heart and blood vessels.

- If needed, take blood pressure pills that can also slow down kidney damage. Two kinds of pills can help:
  - o ACE (angiotensin [an-gee-oh-TEN-sin] converting enzyme inhibitor (in-HIB-it-ur)
  - o ARB (angiotensin receptor blocker)
- Follow the healthy eating plan you work out with your doctor or dietician. If you already have kidney problems, your dietician may suggest that you cut back on protein, such as meat.
- Have your kidneys checked at least once a year by having your urine tested for small amounts of protein.
- Have any other kidney tests that your doctor thinks you need.
- See a doctor for bladder or kidney infections right away if you may have an infection if you have these symptoms:
  - o pain or burning when urinating
  - o frequent urge to urinate
  - o urine that looks cloudy or reddish
  - o fever or shaky feeling
  - o pain in your back or on your side below the ribs

How can my doctor protect my kidneys during special x-ray tests?

If you have kidney damage, the liquid, called a contrast agent, used for special x-ray tests, can make your kidney damage worse. Your doctor can give you extra water before and after the x-ray to protect your kidneys. Or your doctor may order a test that does not use a contrast agent.

How can diabetes hurt my kidneys?

When kidneys are working well, the tiny filters in your kidneys, the glomeruli, keep protein inside your body. You need the protein to stay healthy.

High blood glucose and high blood pressure damage the kidneys' filters. When the kidneys are damaged, the protein leaks out of the kidneys into the urine. Damaged kidneys do not do a good job of cleaning out waste and extra fluids. So, not enough waste and fluids go out of the body as urine. Instead, they build up in your blood.

An early sign of kidney damage is when your kidneys leak small amounts of a protein called albumin (al-BYOO-min) into the urine.

With more damage, the kidneys leak more and more protein. This problem is called proteinuria (PRO-tee-NOOR-ee-uh). More and more wastes build up in the blood. This damage getrs worse until the kidneys fail.

Diabetic nephropathy (neh-FROP-uh-thee) is the medical term for kidney problems caused by diabetes.

How will I know if my kidneys fail?

At first, you cannot tell. Kidney failure from diabetes happens so slowly that you may not feel sick at all for many years. You will not feel sick even when your kidneys do only half the job of normal kidneys. You may not feel any signs of kidney failure until your kidneys have almost stopped working. However, getting your urine and blood checked every year can tell you if your kidneys are not working.

Once your kidneys fail, you may feel sick to your stomach and tired all the time. Your skin may turn yellow. You may feel puffy and your hands and feet may swell from extra fluid in your body.

What happens if my kidneys fail?

First, you will need dialysis (dy-AL-ih-sis) treatment. Dialysis is a treatment that does the work your kidneys used to do. There are two types of dialysis. You and your doctor will decide what type will work best for you. Dialysis is a treatment that takes waste products and extra fluid out of your body.

1. Hemodialysis (HE-mo-dy-AL-ih-sis) In hemodialysis, your blood flows through a tube from your arm to a machine that filters out the waste products and extra fluid. The clean blood flows back to your arm.

2. Peritoneal dialysis (PEH-rih-tuh-NEE-ul dy-AL-ih-sis) In peritoneal dialysis, your belly is filled with a special fluid. The fluid collects waste products and

extra water from your blood. Then the fluid is drained from your body and thrown away.

Second, you may be able to have a kidney transplant. This operation gives you a new kidney. The kidney can be from a close family member, friend, or someone you do not know. You may be on dialysis for a long time. Many people are waiting for new kidneys. A new kidney must be a good match for your body.

Will I know if I start to have kidney problems?

No. You will know if you have kidney problems only if your doctor checks your urine for protein. Do not wait for signs of kidney damage to have your urine checked.

How can I find out if I have kidney problems?

Each year, my doctor checks a sample of my urine to see if my kidneys are leaking small amounts of microalbumin (MY-kro-al-BYOO-min). The test results will tell him how well my kidneys are working.

Other tests can be done to check the kidneys. The doctor might check blood to measure the amounts of creatinine (kree-AT-ih-nin) and urea (yoo-REE-uh). These are waste products our body makes; if the kidneys are not cleaning them out of our blood, they can build up and make us sick.

Your doctor might also ask you to collect your urine in a large container for a whole day or just overnight. Then the urine will be checked for protein.

To determine whether my long-standing diabetes affected

my kidneys, my family physician ordered a laboratory test every year to detect:

- microalbumin
- blood in the urine

Testing my urine is the only way to tell if my body is producing dangerous ketones.

Our body normally uses insulin to convert glucose or sugar to energy. When insulin is not available and our body is unable to convert sugar to energy, it uses fat. When the body does not use fat completely, fat cells break down and produce toxic chemical compounds that make the blood acidic (ketoacidosis). When I want to know whether my urine contains ketones before going to my physician, I buy a self-testing kit from my pharmacy.

How to test for ketones:

1. Dip a Chemstrip K-test strip into a sample of urine. Wait one minute.

2. Compare the test pad color to the color chart on the side of the Chemstrip K-vial.

3. Record the result.

4. Follow the manufacturer's recommendation for care and storage.

Type II non-insulin-dependent diabetics must call their doctor when:

- blood sugar is greater than 240 mg/dl and ketones are positive in urine as shown by the ketones urine test.

- blood sugar has increased over the past 12 hours and the test shows ketones in the urine.

DIABETIC EYE DISEASE (RETINOPATHY)

Retinopathy develops over many years and in several stages. The milder form, background retinopathy, is characterized by leakage and leaks of fluid from capillaries of the retina and swelling that points to eye problems:

- blurry eyesight

- double vision

- vision is distorted or straight lines such as telephone poles look warped

- spots seem to float in front of the eyes

- field of vision seems narrower

- difficulty seeing clearly in dim lights

- feeling pressure or pain in the eyes]

- trouble perceiving color, especially blue and yellow in making distinctions between similar colors.

Capillary breakage and leaks of fluid must have

happened while I was reading a newspaper. Tiny black dots appeared in front of my eyes, blocking my vision. When I looked away, those tiny black dots followed. Wherever I looked, the black dots followed.

To get rid of them, I put eye drops, thinking that my eyes were just tired from too much reading and typing. But while the drops relieved eye fatigue, the tiny dots remained. I was worried.

Suddenly one day while reading the newspaper, everything turned dark. I was terrified.

Frantically I called my ophthalmologist and explained what I was experiencing. He said that my eye blood vessels had hemorrhaged. An emergency appointment was scheduled.

Faces doubled. Images of the same face superimposed on each other. It was weird and shocking.

My ophthalmologist performed laser surgery. He assured me that it would not be painful because the retina does not feel pain. Sure enough. Due to the painkillers, the surgery was not painful. The discomfort came mostly from my fear of the unknown. Even with painkillers, I felt the high-voltage ultra-violet rays bombarding the dilated left eye. I could not even blink because both eyes had to remain dilated.

I wondered why my right eye should not blink when only my left eye was dilated while undergoing surgery. The ophthalmologist knew when my right eye attempted to blink because, in exasperation, he said, "Don't move your eyes. Look straight. LOOK STRAIGHT!" But how? When one eye is undergoing surgery, the other eye is not allowed to even blink or move. Which eye should look straight? The dilated one only? Or both eyes?

He commanded, "Move your eyes to the left."

"Look to the right."

"Look straight ahead."

"Look up."

"Look down."

"Don't blink."

"Keep your eyes wide open." (The eye was dilated and wouldn't close.)

"Keep still."

"Don't move."

"Keep still," when I fidgeted due to the discomfort. "It will only take seven more minutes."

Those seven minutes lasted forever.

After the laser surgery, the ophthalmologist covered my left eye with a soft bandage for a few hours. He prescribed eye drops once a day and scheduled three checkups that year.

After the bandage was removed at home, my left eye dilated while my right eye remained normal. I have no idea when my left eye returned to normal. It did, however, in a matter of hours. When my granddaughter, Aimee, saw me she blurted, OH! Grandma! You look really, honestly weird. What happened?"

Without meaning to, I replied, a little bit annoyed, "Oh, Aimee, please don't look. I'll be normal tomorrow."

The following week, an optician in the same office fitted me with three eyeglasses: one for reading; one for watching TV; and another for protection from the sun.

My ophthalmologist scheduled me for an annual checkup since then.

NERVE DAMAGE (NEUROPATHY)

This chapter includes very useful information pertaining to peripheral nerve damage which the National Information Clearinghouse, National Institute of Health, Department of Health and Human Services recommended be disseminated to the general public.

Here are the instructions on how to prevent diabetes from damaging the nervous system.

Research has shown that people who kept their blood glucose close to normal were able to lower their risk of nerve damage.

- Keep blood glucose as close to normal as possible.

- Limit the amount of alcohol intake.

- Don't smoke.

- Take care of your feet.

- Tell your doctor about any problems noticed with:

  o The hands, arms, feet and legs

  o The stomach, bowels or bladder

  o Tell your doctor about any problems when having sex.

  o Inability to tell when blood glucose is too low

  o Feeling dizzy going from lying down to sitting or standing

What to do to take care of the feet:

- Wash feet in warm water every day. Make sure the water is not too hot by testing the temperature with the elbow. Do not soak feet. Dry feet well, especially between the toes.

- If skin is dry, rub lotion on them after washing. Do not put lotion between the toes.

- Look at feet every day to check for cuts, sores, blisters, redness, calluses or other problems. Checking every day is even more important if one has nerve damage or poor blood flow. If one cannot bend over or pull feet up to check them, use a mirror. If one cannot see well, ask someone else to check the feet.

- File corns and calluses gently with an emery board or pumice stone. Do this after bath or shower.

- Cut toenails once a week when needed. Cut them when they are soft from washing. Cut them to the shape of the toe and not too short. File the edges with an emery board. If you cannot cut your own toenails, ask someone who can or go to a foot doctor.

- Always wear shoes or slippers to protect feet from injuries.

- Always wear socks or stockings to avoid blisters. Do not wear socks or knee-high stockings that are too tight below the knee.

- Wear shoes that fit well. Shop for shoes at the end of the day when your feet are bigger. Break in shoes slowly. Wear them 1 to 2 hours each day for the first 1 to 2 weeks.

- Make sure your doctor checks your feet at each checkup.

What does the nervous system do?

Nerves carry messages back and forth between the brain and other parts of the body. All of our nerves together make up the nervous system.

Some nerves tell the brain what is happening in the body. For example, when we step on a tack, the nerve in our foot tells the brain about the pain. Other nerves tell the body what to do. For example, nerves from the brain tell the stomach when it is time to move food into your intestines.

How can diabetes damage to the peripheral nerves affect us?

Peripheral nerves go to the arms, hands, legs and feet. Damage to these nerves can make our arms, hands, legs or feet feel numb. Also, we might not be able to feel pain, heat or cold when we should. We may feel shooting pains or burning or tingling sensations, like "pins and needles". These feelings are often worse at night. They make it hard to sleep. Most of the time, these feelings are on both sides of your body, like in both feet. But they can be on just one side.

Peripheral nerve damage can change the shape of the feet. Foot muscles get weak and the tendons of the foot get shorter. There are special shoes that are made to fit softly around sore feet that have changed shape. These special shoes help protect the feet. Medicare and other health insurance programs may pay for special shoes. Talk to your doctor about how and where to get these shoes.

How can diabetes damage to the autonomic nerves affect us?

Autonomic nerves help you know that your blood glucose is low. Some people take diabetes medicines that can accidentally make their blood glucose too low. Damage to the autonomic nerves can make it hard for them to feel the symptoms of hypoglycemia (hy-po-gly-SEE-mee-uh), also called low blood glucose.

This kind of damage is more likely to happen if one has

had diabetes for a long time. It can also happen if the blood glucose has been too low very often.

Autonomic nerves go to the stomach, intestines and other parts of the digestive system. Damage to these nerves can make food pass through the digestive system too slowly or too quickly. Nerve problems can cause nausea (feeling sick to your stomach), vomiting, constipation or diarrhea.

Nerve damage to your stomach is called gastroparesis (gas-tro-puh-REE-sis). When nerves to the stomach are damaged, the muscles of the stomach do not work well and food may stay in the stomach too long. Gastroparesis makes it hard to keep blood glucose under control.

Relevant to the issue of nerve damage as it affected me, an article published in *The Star-Ledger* (March 2, 2005) by Dr. Paul G. Donahue of Orlando, Florida wrote that the causes and treatment of neuropathy vary. He defined neuropathy as a nerve disturbance.

According to Dr. Donahue:

"Peripheral nerves are nerves that take messages from the brain and spinal cord and deliver them to muscles and organs—the periphery. Those kinds of nerves are motor nerves. They tell the muscles to contract or glands to secrete. Peripheral nerves also take information from the skin and inner organs and transmit it to the brain. Those are sensory nerves. They inform the brain when something is hurt by transmitting pain. Many nerve cables are a combination of motor and sensory nerves."

'Neuropathy' means there is a nerve disturbance. The consequences can be many. With sensory neuropathy, people can lose all sensation or, more commonly, they can have persistent and severe pain. The pain is described as burning, freezing, knifelike or similar to an electric shock. When motor nerves are affected, muscles become weak. One sign is foot weakness. Peripheral neuropathy of the muscles can make them so weak that they cannot lift the foot when taking a step.

Symptoms of both kinds of neuropathy can remain stationary for long periods or they can progress rapidly and incapacitate people.

Treatment depends on cause, and causes are many. Diabetes often leads to peripheral neuropathy. An assault on nerves by the immune system is another somewhat-common cause. A few infections can cause neuropathies. The pain that lasts after a shingles attack is an example. In some parts of the world, vitamin deficiencies are the major cause. Some neuropathies are genetically induced. Quite often, however, no cause is found.

A large number of medicines can be helpful for pain relief. Gabapentin, amitriptyline, lidocaine skin patches and Zostrix cream are examples. Cymbalta and Lyrica are newly-approved drugs for diabetic neuropathy. They should be available soon, if they are not on the market at this writing. Occupational and physical therapists can provide programs and devices that help people with motor neuropathy to overcome muscle malfunction.

For years,

1. I felt burning, tingling, painful sensations in both feet. My legs and toes seemed to have tiny bugs crawling inside the skin.

2. My two hands felt pain and stiffness right up to my elbows.

3. I suffered from painful, restless legs.

4. My skin was itchy, dry, rough and sensitive as if it would tear off.

5. I suffered frequent bronchitis, coughs, colds, runny eyes, runny nose, mild fever and chills whenever the weather changed.

6. My fingernails and toenails constantly broke so much that they developed hard calluses.

7. I had pain in my arms and elbows; breaking fingernails and toenails and burning sensation in legs and feet.

My diabetic specialist said, "All these symptoms could subside or lessen with good blood sugar control, exercise and medication." Yet even with my daily blood tests showing acceptable sugar levels of 110 to130 mg/dl, the physical discomfort and painful sensations continued.

Painkillers allowed me to sleep, but the side effect was drowsiness and grouchiness at work and with my family.

Leg cramps often accompanied the burning and tingling.

Occasionally I relieved them with rubbing alcohol, mineral ice, Icy Hot, Biofreeze cream or tourniquets.

So much pain in both hands up to the elbows caused extreme difficulty in washing my hair or cooking. I couldn't even hold pots and pans, coffee cups, plates or even spoons and forks. I felt crippled.

My family physician referred me to a hand, arm and forearm specialist.

This specialist diagnosed this as carpal tunnel syndrome.

The Merck Manual of Medical Information defines Carpal Tunnel Syndrome as "a compression of the median nerve that travels through the wrist supporting the thumb which produces numbness, tingling, pain and burning sensations in the arms and shoulders. This condition is common among women whose work requires repeated forceful movement such as typing and using the computer. Carpal Tunnel Syndrome is common with diabetics and with those having an underactive thyroid.

The specialist put braces (splints) on my arms and hands to relieve pressure. While the braces were on, I had no pain at all. But the aches and pains returned as soon as the braces were removed. The pain traveled to my elbow. I could not comb my hair. I could not use forks or spoons or wash my face. The specialist suggested cortisone injections to combat the inflammation. I could not agree without a second opinion.

Understanding my predicament, my family physician

suggested a different hand and forearm orthopedic surgeon.

The second orthopedic surgeon prescribed two months of physical rehabilitation at Bayshore Community Hospital. This therapy consisted of running an electrical current on my arms and shoulder, followed by up-and-down, left-and-right motions as if I were doing karate exercises at home twice daily.

After two months, the aches and pains in my arms, wrist and elbow subsided. But two months later the pain suddenly jolted me from sleep. What did I do wrong this time?

I went back to the second orthopedic surgeon. He requested copies of physical examinations, tests and medications given by the hospital and by my family physician.

This second orthopedic surgeon prescribed low-level *OXYCONTIN* tablets once or twice daily if needed for pain when it was so severe that I could not rest or sleep at all.

However, a controversy about over-prescribing Oxycontin to Rush Limbaugh that led to his famous drug abuse issue scared me too much to take Oxycontin. But since I was in such excruciating pain, I took it anyway.

WAS IT POWERFUL!! Just one tablet made me very calm and pain-free and in a happy, singing mood.

Fortunately, the Oxycontin did not make me dizzy, drowsy or lethargic. It temporarily erased all distress and physical pain as if by magic. I felt I could not only face the world and tackle my work with a smile, but still function efficiently at home. But only while its effect had not worn off. Ten days later I craved Oxycontin even after taking the prescribed one tablet or two daily as needed.

I got irritable and grouchy when I did not give in to the craving. I became restless and could not sleep. I stopped taking Oxycontin right then and went through a short, very painful withdrawal. I am grateful to have detected my susceptibility to this addictive medication. It could have caused me a lot of trouble.

Immediately I informed the second orthopedic surgeon about my stopping the Oxycontin. He suggested three cortocortizoid injections to my elbow. "If those injections fail, you should have surgery. Your excessive pain is due to a dislocated shoulder blade.

Now I was really scared. The first orthopedic surgeon diagnosed carpal tunnel syndrome. The second diagnosed a dislocated shoulder blade. How could this be? The physical therapist at Bayshore Community Hospital manipulated my shoulder by moving my arms left and right, up and down and sidewise with no pain at all. I did the same exercises at home. The excruciating pain was from my right elbow – not from my shoulder blade.

I told my husband I would live with my pain with over-the-counter painkillers. I would not submit to surgery until three specialists agreed on the same cause.

When my family physician heard of my decision he prescribed Tylenol with codeine only when extremely necessary, like when sleep became impossible. He also gave me Naproxen tablets and liniment rub. I tried Icy Hot; Mineral Ice; Bengay; Aspercreme. The newspapers and TV News reported Naproxen (Aleve) can lead to death. I stopped taking Naproxen without telling my doctor.

I continued using liniment rubs when the pain was unbearable until after 2003, one year after I had been taking "the food" – a can of baby's milk – which became my means of solving all these nagging body aches and pains.

RESTLESS LEG SYNDROME

Studies published by *The New York Times* and by *The Star-Ledger* in 2004 claimed that a team of doctors from the University of Medicine and Dentistry of New Jersey and from the Robert Wood Johnson Medical School, also of New Jersey, as well as by physicians from Montreal, Canada and Milan, Italy concluded that Restless Leg Syndrome is a neurological disorder manifested by uncontrollable urges to move the legs to the point of disrupting sleep and interfering with daily lives. It also concluded, "This disorder often goes unrecognized because many doctors fail to recognize it."

No wonder! From 1994 to 2001 the cause of the uncontrollable movements of my legs when at rest was not accurately determined.

My symptoms pertaining to restless leg syndrome included:

- pain in the legs and a sensation that tiny bugs were crawling inside my skin

- extreme discomfort, especially when at rest, sitting and lying down

- strange sensations of numbness accompanied by uncomfortable and uncontrollable leg jerkings up-and-down and sidewise.

I often had to get out of bed and massage my legs with hot compresses, then rub liberal amounts of Mineral Ice or Icy Hot for temporary relief.

Nothing mentioned in these newly-released studies indicated that Restless Leg Syndrome is caused by diabetes. Yet it is my personal observation that when my blood sugar rose higher than 200 mg/dl, both my legs felt numb and ready to jerk whether seated, standing or at rest. The jerkings and kicking started mildly at first and then became violent.

The single cause noted by these studies is neurological disorder. *NEUROLOGICAL DISORDER!!* Was something wrong with my brain cells? Was I suffering from mental health issues?

Goodness! How scary!

GOD FORBID!!

Again, my family physician advised me to apply hot compresses or mineral ice. When these were not enough, he changed my prescription to two 250 mg Aleve tablets. Again! I did not order the prescription (Naproxen). To calm my nerves and help me sleep, he also prescribed .50 mg Xanax, which made me drowsy and sleepy day and night.

Taking Xanax for over six months made my conversation incoherent and my speech slurred.

One of my cousins, a nurse, said that perhaps I was over-medicated.

Desperately, my husband recommended chiropractic treatment, which consisted of:

- twice-a-week electronic massages on my legs and lumbar
- massages of mineral ice or other liniment before bed

Chiropractic seemed to work. My legs responded positively. But a year after I stopped, the restlessness of both legs returned, along with pain and swelling of my ankles. These caused walking difficulties.

We consulted yet another specialist who recommended X-rays and an MRI, both of which had been done before. This latest specialist claimed that the pain in my knees was fluid buildup due to the onset of rheumatoid arthritis. He suggested arthroscopic surgery to take out the fluid in the legs. As before, I refused.

The last specialist that we consulted examined the restlessness of my legs, the pain in my knees and swelling in my ankles. He diagnosed fibromyalgia syndrome, since I limped stiff with pain. Like other specialists before, he also recommended painkillers or surgery if they did not work.

But by this time, I no longer believed that any pain medication would work. Those painkillers merely deadened my senses but provided no healing. What other medication could he prescribe? Sensing my thought, he prescribed drugs similar to those that were given in the past like Motrin or Aleve, but with stronger doses of 500 mg – double the usual 250 mg. Again, the prescription was merely pain killers which dulled my senses temporarily but provided no cure.

I resigned myself to a life of tortured pain and a bleak future with crutches or a cane. Or, worse of all, paralysis.

In 2003, my very dismal outlook changed radically and unbelievably.

I attribute this to a simple can of baby's milk.

CHAPTER V

How Baby's Milk Healed My Diabetes Nerve Damage and Physical Aches and Pain

In October, 2002, my daughter asked me to take care of my three-month-old grandson. I was surprised because her original plan was to hire a professional babysitter, but she feared entrusting Little Matthew's care to one after she saw news about babysitters abusing babies by hitting, slapping and shoving them. Since I saw the same news report, how could I refuse?

I agreed immediately, without taking into consideration my illness and my age and the efforts it takes to take care of an ever-growing infant.

Sure enough, when Little Matthew, at six months, became colicky and cried and writhed in pain, it seemed as if he would slip from my arms as I tried to pacify him. It was difficult to hold him and press him to my tummy to ease his pain by the warmth from my body since my two arms were too painful to lift him as well as I should. The gas pain drops prescribed for him did not take effect until a few minutes later. When the gas pain subsided, he did not want to be lowered into his crib; he was scared and wanted to be held for comfort. I was scared for his safety each morning before he arrived. But I could not tell anyone. I became attached to him immediately. I remember, too, that his mom had planned to give up working instead of hiring a stranger to baby-sit, should I be unable to help.

A very good-paying job which my daughter has is very hard to find. I didn't want her to stop working. I decided right then that I would double the amount of painkillers I took to dull my pain. This way I could hold the baby very carefully so there'd be no possibility of him slipping from my arms. I even tied a white cloth around my neck like a small hammock to support little Matthew to sleep when he did not want to stay in his crib. It worked.

One day while feeding Baby Matthew his ready-made liquid-milk formula in his sixth month, I observed how strong, healthy, bright-eyed and cheerful he had grown since. Despite the colic, his grip was strong as he held my fingers. His arms and legs constantly kicked and flapped as he cooed and smiled. His bright and animated eyes reacted to the sunlight from the window and to the hanging musical toys above the crib.

Baby's milk is the life force that develops cells, nerves and vital organs of babies in their first year. Baby's milk in either liquid, ready-to-feed formula or powdered milk in the can is a good substitute for mother's milk. My five children, all adults, grew healthy on it.

As I observed Matthew's growth week after week, I wondered: would baby's formula regenerate, rejuvenate, re-grow the cells, glands, body organs and blood vessels in my sickly, aching body?

Preposterous! No doctor ever suggested using baby's formula the way I was imagining and/or thinking.

But the seemingly "preposterous" idea nagged me.

Alone with Little Matthew eleven hours a day with little else to do when he was asleep, the "preposterous" idea kept bothering me while sleeping and while awake.

Although I drink coffee with milk every day, I have never drunk infant ready-made liquid milk formula. However, many years ago, I shared my children's powdered milk by diluting it with water when I was fatigued, but never regularly.

Since the "preposterous" idea kept nagging me, I thought to self-experiment. Since no other person would be involved, I gave in to my idea, just hoping for the best.

One day when I went food shopping, I bought a ready-to-use liquid infant formula. A 13-ounce can cost only $4.98, which I consumed in two days, since I only drank 3 ounces two times a day at first. I was cautious at the start. I continued taking the liquid infant formula for ten months.

A year later, I changed to powdered infant milk of the same brand. A 25.7-ounce and a 28.5-ounce can cost only $23.98. I have consumed this powdered infant milk every day, diluted with water, according to the directions on the label. I drank six ounces of this milk three times a day for a total of 18 ounces daily.

Milk is healthy, but compared with liquid infant milk, would infant powdered milk produce the same positive results for adults and much more for an elderly, physically-deteriorating diabetic like me?

The nutritional contents of Matthew's baby milk either in liquid or powdered form are perfect for a growing child. It has complete nutritional content on which babies grow. The formula contained 4,614 calories per five fluid ounces. Matthew drank five fluid ounces five times daily, or six times when needed. I was allowed only 1800 calories per day in my diet plan.

Would I be taking too much risk with six ounces of powdered milk diluted with water three times daily? Would three ounces of liquid formula which contained about 2,742 calories also be too much, considering my meal plan in 2002 was for only 1800 calories per day?

Well, what was my alternative? I was not getting better physically, and I was getting more depressed and demoralized each day from the unexplained physical pain.

I resolved to proceed with my self-experiment. If my blood glucose became dangerously elevated due to the nutritional content in baby's milk, I would rush to the emergency room and stop the experiment. I had nothing to lose.

Was it insight? Inspiration? Helplessness? Abiding faith? that made me self-experiment?

Intrigued and hopeful, when my husband and I went food shopping, I copied the nutritional contents of several ready-to-use liquid infant formulas. At home I typed all the information to find out whether different brands of liquid baby formula have similar ingredients and nutritional contents compared to powdered one. I found very minimal difference.

However, despite almost similar nutritional contents, I found to my utter surprise that different brands have different tastes and different smells. Some caused me hyperacidity; a couple cause me diarrhea.

I self-experimented with the brand that Baby Matthew was taking. The medicinal taste and smell of the ready-to-use liquid formula turned me off. I had to add a few drops of vanilla extract to swallow it. I still had to hold my nose because of the very strong smell that stayed on my breath all day. The aftertaste proved intolerable.

It took me months to adjust to the indescribable medicinal taste and smell. Still, I resolved to keep taking the same formula. My grandson took to this formula like it was the most natural enjoyable food in the world. Of course, he knew no other taste and no other smell.

After taking Matthew's ready-to-feed formula for six months, I looked for a liquid formula that is pleasant to the taste and with minimal medicinal smell. I realized that the multi-vitamin content of the liquid formula caused the medicinal taste. I lucked out when I found a ready-to-feed formula with no aftertaste and very mild, which did not cause me high acidity. I stayed with this ready-to-feed liquid formula for six additional months. When Little Matthew was fifteen months old, I switched to the powdered form of this other milk with no medicinal taste. I have continued taking this other milk in powdered form to this day.

My Food Exchange Meal Plan is a diet plan for diabetics. It allowed me only 1800 calories per day. Therefore, I was hungry most of the time. Even when I had half a cup of coffee with low-fat milk and unsalted crackers at snack time (twice daily), I was hungry still.

Since taking the powdered milk diluted with water according to instructions on the can made me feel full, I did not crave snacks between meals. This helped me maintain my doctor's approved weight of 110-120 lbs for my height of 5'2".

POSITIVE BENEFITS OF MY EXPERIMENTS WITH BABY'S MILK

1. My brittle fingernails no longer break and do not look ugly and unkempt.

Within six months of taking the baby's ready-made liquid formula followed by the powdered formula, the nails in my hands and feet stopped breaking. They grew soft, strong and clean-looking; free of yellowish, brownish discoloration like cigarette tar. Manicuring and pedicuring them is now a joy.

2. The painful swelling of my knuckles and finger joints is also gone.

Today, I can manipulate and bend my fingers, close and open them, which I was unable to do for years. I can now write legibly and type my papers. I can button my clothes;

open soda bottles and jars of pickles; close and open closet doors with no pain. The tremors in my hands when under so much stress and pain disappeared too.

3. The calluses and cracks on my feet and around my cuticles have healed.

Nail cutting is no longer painful and dangerous. The softening of cuticles has made pedicuring easy. I can now bend at my waistline to cut my toenails and do manicure and pedicure, which I wasn't able to do for years.

Most of all, bending when doing chores and when exercising is no longer painful and difficult.

4. The hands and arms that I could not lift, once-diagnosed with carpal tunnel syndrome, onset of arthritis, shoulder blade dislocation, I can now raise, lower turn sidewise and rotate.

I AM NOW PAIN-FREE!

Best of all, I can lift and carry twenty-eight-month-old Matthew when he raises his arms, which is often. I can follow him with little difficulty when he runs around the house. I can play ball and even walk around the block with him.

But in the past, when we played throwball and the small ball slipped from my hands or I failed to throw the ball back to him, puzzlement was all over his face.

Startled and frustrated, Matthew used to run toward me, his two tiny arms outstretched and flailing, mouthing garbled unintelligible words demonstrating for me to throw the ball, saying "'ere! (Here!) 'Ere, Gamma, look my 'and (hand)", gesturing me to throw or catch a ball.

In 2005 he was almost three years old, a very nice, energetic, sweet young boy* who says, "Thank you," "I love you," and seldom keeps still. Of course, he seldom walks; he prefers to run, skip and jump as if to tease me while he squeals with laughter as I remind him, "Walk slowly. Walk slowly." As I follow him merrily everywhere without the usual nagging pain in my joints, it is humbling when a young child who is beginning to speak tries to teach an adult. He trusted me. He felt I was his playmate. When the playmate could not do what he could, he felt let down, gave up and chose toys he could play with quietly alone or with me. His perception of adult situations without fussing still puts lumps in my throat.

5. My chafed, flaky, dried and itchy rough skin on my face, arms, legs and neckline began to smooth, with wrinkles on them greatly diminished.

Pharmacists and physicians' recommended moisturizers which I have applied all over my skin to ease the dryness and itchiness have only provided temporary softness to my very dry, rough skin, after which the same problems recurred.

---

*Matthew turned 7 in June, 2009.

These moisturizers were multi-vitamin-based; milk-based; lanolin-based. Some were moisturizing rich soaps such as Dove, Lever 2000, Oilatum, Neutrogena and Aveeno. Still others were Aveeno Cream, Cortizone Plus Créme, Aquapor Créme and even Epilyt Oil – every skin moisturizer in the United States.

I used them all.

However, I found the Aquapor Créme and Aveeno Anti-Itch Cream to be two of the most effective in relieving the itchiness and dryness of my skin, but again, only temporarily. I have applied either one at least four times a day.

While I lay no blame on any skin emollient, I could not understand why my abhorrent skin condition was not alleviated by any of them.

There was no healing either inside or outside my skin until 2003, when, gradually, the flakiness and roughness very much diminished within six months after taking a simple can of baby milk – which I refer to here as "the food". The hydration, youthfulness, softening and smoothness of my skin with diminished wrinkles I attribute to the baby's milk which no cosmetics had effectively done.

6. Frequent upper respiratory problems such as chronic bronchitis, runny eyes, runny nose, flu-like general discomfort, frequent sneezing, sore throats, coughing and chills have disappeared.

Even though I received flu shots in early October of each

year, they did not prevent the recurrence of upper respiratory problems at each change in the weather or seasons.

Respiratory problems started with runny eyes, runny nose, tiredness, back and muscle aches. Since these conditions had recurred a minimum of four times a year, I have learned to carefully monitor them.

When the early chills, runny eyes, runny nose and sore throat failed to respond to salt and lemon juice gargle, lozenges, hot tea with lemon, Tylenol Flu, Claritin and Zyrtex, I knew from experience that coughs would follow and that bronchitis would start.

In the past, most of these ailments responded positively to Sugar Free Robitussin, Sugar Free Cough Syrup or Brometaine with no sugar. However, when persistent coughing and mild fever lasted seven days, my family physician prescribed cold and cough medicine with codeine to help me sleep, and nose and nasal sprays like Flonase, Claritin, Zyrtex or Allegra. He expected the symptoms to be cured in a week, but when the respiratory obstruction was severe, he prescribed antibiotics like amoxicillin. A nurse at his office surmised that my recurring illness was because diabetics and older people have more difficulty even with strong antibiotics due to a decreased immune system.

Amoxicillin usually cleared my bronchial problems. When I complained of chest pains and the usual X-rays were taken, the emergency room doctor assured me that the pain was caused by persistent coughing and sneezing and not by mini-stroke.

Promethazine with Codeine was the usual prescription given to ease the chest pain and to give relief for rest and sleep. The most potent antibiotic given to me was Zythromax (Z-pak) which, my experience indicated, is not a mere painkiller but strongly helped more than any other medication in alleviating my recurring upper respiratory problems within 7 days.

Yet even with the potent Zythromax, my respiratory problems continued with every season change, which I dreaded.

I have been spared the regular three to four dangerous attacks to my respiratory system since 2004, 11 months after I experimented with "the food" – a simple can of baby's milk.

In the Spring of 2003, I had a few sniffles or mild colds, but the severe bronchial problems did not again torture me. In the Fall and Winter of 2004, flu vaccine was not available in many parts of the United States due to bacteria contamination in the laboratories of the major U.S. suppliers in the United Kingdom. As a result, I am one who did not receive flu vaccine.

In spite of the fact that I did not receive flu immunization in 2004, the flu-like symptoms that chronically attached me for 14 years have not returned.

I continue having flu vaccine each year as a preventive measure.

Recent X-rays showed very clear lungs, very well-functioning kidneys, normal blood pressure and a good cholesterol level.

My blood sugar? Acceptable. Neither too high nor too low to cause alarm.

The advent of 2005 is clearly a joyous year for me health-wise.

In less than two years after taking the baby's milk, my skin no longer itches. It looks and feels soft, plumped and hydrated. Wrinkles on my forehead, bridge of my nose, corners of my mouth, eyes and neckline greatly cleared and diminished. The baby's ready-to-feed liquid formula and powdered baby's milk brought about these positive changes of making my skin respond from the inside, which no cosmetics had effectively done for me.

In 2005, our young neighbors, in their early thirties, came to our front yard where my husband was weeding. They invited us to their barbecue that afternoon. We had to decline because we were attending a party at my 44-year-old daughter's, also that afternoon.

Amazed, our neighbor exclaimed, *"You have a 44-year-old daughter?"*

We all laughed.

"Yes," I answered, "you two could be the same ages of my other younger children."

We all laughed again.

My husband gazed at me. "Yes, doesn't she look great!

Nida, do you believe me now?" Often he had commented that I looked much, much better lately, but I shrugged my shoulders when he said it, thinking he was only flattering me. (Just like a man.)

This spontaneous compliment was the best I received from a man young enough to be my son. The compliments from him and from my husband made my day then. They make my day now.

It seemed that their compliments went to my head. That afternoon I scrutinized my face in the bathroom mirror and in a hand-held mirror to see for myself. The two mirrors showed me a face with very much diminished wrinkles. I went to bed smiling.

7. My restless legs have calmed down.

My two legs that felt numbed, prickly and which kicked/thrashed violently at rest have calmed down. Occasionally, one or both legs felt so numb and tense that it seemed they would violently move.

But massaging them with my hands pressing against the muscles kept the muscles still. Once in a while I felt cramps in one leg. Again, holding down the muscles kept them under control. I have not had restless legs kicking violently since 2005, over a year and a half since taking the baby's formula.

8. There has been a dramatic increase in my physical stamina and ability to sustain energy.

While previously I had difficulties doing household

chores, all that has changed. I can cook and clean while young Matthew sleeps. Now, I can put clothes in the washer and dryer and sweep the kitchen floor. Best of all, I can play with Matthew without wincing in pain.

For example, I blew bubbles for him to chase. In the past, I could not blow my birthday candles out. Either I did not have enough strength or I lacked oxygen in my system. Matthew and I also chased butterflies the summer of 2004 and took walks around Hazlet. We also waited at the street corner for Aimee to get out of the yellow bus when she came home from school.

9. Now I can take long walks with no pain. I can even dance socially and wear low-heeled leather shoes.

Were it not for my new stamina and vitality, it would be impossible to push Matthew in the driveway and around the block as he rides his cart when he does not wish to walk; to continue caring daily for this energetic, happy young child who climbs and slides on furniture, who seldom keeps still when awake; who jumps on chairs and tabletops Tarzan-style.

March 13, 2004, my husband and I attended my cousin Linda's retirement party. I ate (in moderation, of course) every food in the buffet: Italian-American; Chinese; Filipino, including summer fruits and sweets against which my diet plan warned me. When I tested my blood sugar at home, there was no dangerously high glucose. The reading was 141 mg/dl: still under acceptable glucose level.

Considering that I deviated from my food exchange plan, it amazed me that my blood sugar did not shoot up like it used to before I took the baby's milk. Considering all the forbidden food I took, could the result of my blood test be wrong?

I did it again the following week when my daughter took me to dinner at an Italian restaurant. I consumed more than during Linda's retirement because the food was so good and so appetizing and also to test whether my glucose level would be highly elevated as a result.

When I tested it two hours after returning home, the glucose level was a little bit higher, 160 mg/dl. I was so elated because while the glucose level was high, it was not dangerously high and which could be remedied by better management of my diet or food intake. After a few more deviations from my food exchange plan, the test results varied from 120 mg/dl -137 mg/dl, all under acceptable levels. I realized that I could give up the hospital-made food exchange plan and replace it with a food plan of my own, which I did.

I became less strict with my diet but careful of my food intake. My food has little salt; absolutely no sugar; and food fried in very little oil is drained and allowed to dry on paper napkins.

I refrained from red meat most days. On occasions when I had to have red meat for its protein value, I only have a slice about ½ inch thick, thin-sliced pork tenderloin, beefsteak or flank steak. Giving up the hospital-made food exchange plan and following the 2200 calorie meal plan approved by my physician did not mean I threw caution to the winds. Over a decade the food exchange plan instilled the habit of counting calories. It is as I am still on it. The difference is that I became less strict with my diet. I no longer measure my food intake by spoons or tablespoons or grams of fat. When I want two medium-sized cups of vegetables, I have them without worrying that I am overeating.

I can now have four tablespoons of white rice instead of only one. Occasionally I indulge in Chinese food, choosing foods that have no sauce or has no sugar, a nectarine or an apple and small bowl of other fruits without counting the calorie content and feeling horribly guilty.

I now feel like a human being instead of like a small bird that keeps eating tiny bits of grain. All these good feelings I attribute to the baby's milk that made me feel whole and not sick any more.

In addition, at my cousin Linda's retirement, for the first time in a decade I wore Italian leather shoes with 1½ inch heels completely free of pain. My beige shoes complementing my reddish suit and handbag made me feel like the belle of the party over a sea of people wearing dark black attire.

I even waltzed!

IMAGINE!

At first my legs felt stiff. Then gradually I noted the

absence of muscle pain. My legs felt light and my feet glided like when I was young. It felt very good.

Was I simply imagining my youth? It was awe-inspiring and spiritually uplifting to feel how good life had become since I took the baby's milk.

Three months later, in June, 2004, my husband and I stayed overnight at the Trump Plaza Hotel and Casino in Atlantic City. That evening we walked two miles hand-in-hand slowly along the boardwalk before dinner. Although my legs felt tired, there was no pain at all.

Usually, at night when my legs are either tired or at rest, they kick violently and uncontrollably. It did not happen. I slept deeply that night.

The next morning after an early breakfast, we walked the other side of the boardwalk as far as my legs would tolerate, resting every few minutes on the benches facing the Atlantic Ocean.

We enjoyed the morning breeze as we watched cyclists riding on the boardwalk and birds gliding overhead.

My lungs filled with fresh air from the ocean. The cool morning breeze got warmer with the rising sun hugging my whole being, filling me with warmth. I feel cold most of the time, even in summer. To feel warm without the help of a jacket on this particular day was a gift.

"We'll do this again, a few more times this summer," my husband promised.

Since 2005, we have been visiting and walking the boardwalk of Atlantic City twice a year in the Summer and Fall. We also visited Niagara Falls in 2006 where I walked back and forth twice from the American Falls to the Canadian Falls just to test whether my legs would hold.

My legs and my physical stamina were further tested by the long walks we experienced along the dusty very rugged unpaved roads of Ancient Rome in 2007 including visits to medieval cathedrals and the ruins and exploration of Pompeii, destroyed by Mount Vesuvius. There was a heat wave during our visit in 2007. Yet my legs and physical energy remained high even though I felt famished and thirsty for a glass of orange juice or cold water that turned warm due to extreme heat.

My stamina continued to support the unbelievable long walks and climb up to the Arc de Triomphe and long walks over three days along the Champs Elysees with short rests between benches under the shade of the trees where I observed cavernous moss-covered buildings and wondered why people are attracted to the city of Paris and the Palace of Versailles' guilded perhaps by actual gold when there are no cafes and ladies' room facilities for tourists.

My legs that usually are having muscle spasms when tired, continued to cooperate on the hilly climb and pink cobbled stone walks in Monaco and in the south of France, surrounded by the blue water of the Mediterranean that turned deep indigo, as my eyes wandered its expanse.

This sustained energy could not be due to the so-called

Mediterranean diet of oversized servings of green, leafy vegetables and tomatoes and olive oil and french fries and fried breaded fish with wine---foods that are overloaded with carbohydrates which diabetics have been warned not to overindulge. (Read the New Glucose Revolution 2009.)

I am sure the baby's milk which I carried with me during all my trips and which I ingested made me feel full all day held me from overindulging in those rich, nutritious foods.

It was so good to feel alive once again, to feel that life was getting better and worth living. Had it not been for the baby's milk, would I feel the "gift of life" again? Would I feel re-energized and what seemed my slowly-ebbing life revived?

Not a chance. Since 1993 I had been drained of energy. I lived in fear of dying sooner than the long, healthy life I've prayed for.

Taking the baby's milk gave me much more hope than I ever felt possible.

During my recent consultation, I wondered aloud to our family physician, Dr. Thomas Scuderi, whether I could stop diabetic pills. I felt well.

This very kind, most caring doctor warned, "Feeling as if you are no longer diabetic is an illusion. You will always have diabetes."

"Diabetes is for life. It has no cure. You must always observe the regimen of a healthy diet, daily exercise and continue taking your prescribed diabetic pills twice daily," he admonished. "And keep testing your blood sugar. Make sure your readings are on acceptable levels."

I did not tell him about my self-experiment with the baby's milk nor the new menu I made based on the glycemic food written in the glucose revolution books. I followed his advice of taking medication and exercise like a bible.

Despite the positive changes in the quality of my life, the reality is that I will always have diabetes.

In spite of this painful reality, I feel alive; more alive than in years. I no longer feel depressed and useless. I have been feeling very well and, illusion or not, I believe I received an extension of life to enjoy free of physical pain. I can continue nurturing my young grandson who inspired me to self-experiment and to write about my experience with his baby's milk.

I sincerely believe that the positive changes in my life came because of the baby's milk which I am still taking.

I swear that the baby's milk healed the nerve damage that caused me untold pain and torture for 14 years hopefully will prevent it from recurring.

Milk is a complete food that builds up cells, provides immunity from diseases and ensures growth and calms the nerves of babies and adults – as my experience illustrates.

Could people 30 years and older, even though they are not diabetic but stressed, benefit from baby's milk?

Yes, I believe so. Baby's milk is healthy. It does not cause high blood pressure; it does not elevate cholesterol; it does not clog kidneys with toxins; it calms the nerves and reduces stress.

Baby's milk is easily affordable since it costs less than a cheeseburger; less than an anti-depressant; less than pain-killers; less than alcohol; less than cigarettes.

As I said before, my recent tests and X-rays this year 2009 showed very clear lungs; very well-functioning kidneys; normal blood pressure and a good cholesterol level. Is there a better food than baby's milk?

Does one have to be diabetic with nerve damage to benefit from the baby's milk? Not necessarily, in my opinion.

Can non-diabetics benefit? Certainly.

The United States Congress wants more neuropathy research and has directed the National Institute for Neurological Disorders and Strokes (NINDS) to develop a neuropathy research agenda. It would be wonderful if practitioners, scientists and researchers heeded this call and replicate my baby's milk experiment. Would the National Institute of Health provide funds?

The results of my experiment clearly indicate that nutrients in baby's milk could be the keys to the Fountain of Youth. Food and Cosmetic Laboratories around the world could help millions of youth-obsessed people realize a wonderful dream of looking young and youthful turn to reality.

As I said before, since taking baby's milk, my skin has plumped and hydrated, leaving my forehead, corners of my eyes, mouth and neckline with diminished wrinkles. The baby's milk worked from inside my skin, which no cosmetics were able to do for me.

The positive effects that the baby's milk brought about in my physical appearance are obvious to my friends and family and as I look and compare how my face appeared in:

- my unretouched 1987 picture attached to my Naturalization Certificate when I was 49 years old (Federal rules prohibit copying)

- My unretouched non-driver photo ID Issued by the New Jersey Motor Vehicles Office in 2007

The contrast in my facial appearance is very obvious.

In 1984 at age 49, I looked sick, aged.

At age 69, in my 2007 non-drivers photo ID from the Motor Vehicles Office – I look younger, more energetic and healthier which many people my age would love to look. I wanted to show my 2007 photo ID, but federal and state laws prohibit it. Just go to this book's back cover to see how I look at age 72 as a result of drinking baby's milk.

All these physical improvements in my appearance and positive attitude I attribute to the baby's milk I am still taking.

In 2002, at almost 62 years old, I agreed to take care of my grandson, Matthew, whom I still take care of after school.

At present, at almost 72 years old, I'm taking care of three grandchildren. Where did I get the energy and stamina? I have no doubt it's from the baby's milk.

If my health and energy level hold, due to the baby's milk, in my 80's I might sky-dive from an airplane. (Just kidding.)

But who knows?

This could be my last adventure before facing the sunset of my life.

CONCLUSION

I am writing this personal story because I am so grateful to return to a life without the chronic physical and mental pain that so gravely impacted my life for over eighteen years.

It is my hope that readers suffering similarly debilitating sudden fluctuations of blood glucose and diabetic nerve damage shall find equally similar hope and inspiration from my personal experience.

I believe in THE HANDS that show me many miracles: the return of my health, energy, stamina and hope for a very long life.

To me, I received a miracle in this solution to my pain. I hope that my personal experience will enable others to also find their miracles.

However, since I am not a medical practitioner, I can neither give advice nor endorse a baby's milk.

Although taking a baby's milk made very positive changes from my former dark world of daily pain and illness to my present world of sunshine and pure joy of living, my experience may have varied results for others.

I cannot mention the brand name and producer of the baby's milk I experimented on. I am not endorsing any particular baby's milk.

I merely share my happy, positive experience.

Anyone may adapt what I did, anywhere.

Readers must consult their doctor for advice and monitor themselves carefully.

Nevertheless, my experimentation with baby's milk and with low-glucose foods paid off handsomely in many unimaginable ways.

As a result of my newfound good health, I have returned to the pursuit of goals I gave up, like writing; re-establishing a business; planting food crops and trees in my farm in the Philippines and traveling to other countries I have never seen, as well as visiting different places in the United States and Canada.

All these physical improvements in my appearance and positive attitude I attribute to the baby's milk I am still taking and having found solutions to the abrupt fluctuations of my insulin level.

ABOUT THE AUTHOR

Mrs. Leonida Lidman received an M.A. in Education from the University of The Philippines and an M.S. in Human Resources Management from the New School for Social Research, New School University, Fifth Avenue, New York City, in 1987.

She also graduated in 2009 with an advanced writing course from The Long Ridge Writers' Group School, Long Ridge, West Redding, Connecticut.

Her work experiences include being a college instructor in the Philippines; Training Supervisor for Comprehensive Community Health Programs at the University of The Philippines, Bay, Los Baños, Laguna. She also served as Commissioner of the Newark Senior Citizens Commission and Program Coordinator for the Office on Aging, Newark Housing Authority, in Newark N.J. from 1987 to 1989. She was a City Council President's awardee for distinguished community service on behalf of the city's elderly.

She has also written various articles and is a published author.

She is also a recipient of U.S. Patent #4,680,179, a fruit-flavored coconut water-based liqueur with no added sugar and no preservatives.

She has also done volunteer work with the Executive Planning Committee of The United Way, Essex County, New

Jersey and coordinated the recruitment of retired senior volunteers (RSVP Program) for the New Jersey Department of Community Affairs, Essex County, New Jersey and others.

www.ingramcontent.com/pod-product-compliance
Lightning Source LLC
Chambersburg PA
CBHW031215270326
41931CB00006B/568